Conservation genetics of endangered horse breeds

The EAAP series is published under the direction of Dr. P. Rafai

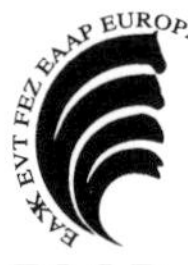

EAAP – European Association for Animal Production

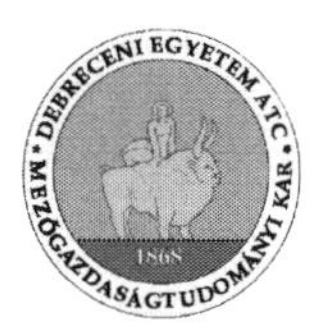

Univesity of Debrecen

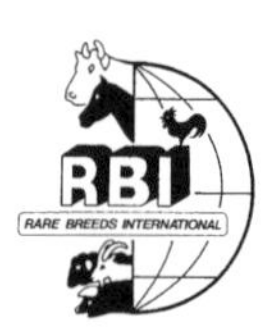

Rare Breeds International

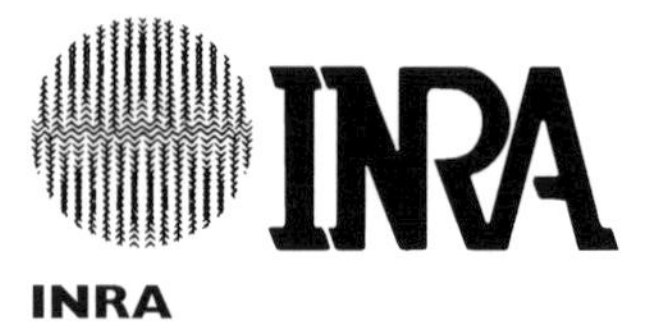

INRA

The European Association for Animal Production wishes to express its appreciation to the *Ministero per le Politiche Agricole e Forestali* and the *Associazione Italiana Allevatori* for their valuable support of its activities

Conservation genetics of endangered horse breeds

EAAP publication No. 116

Editors:

Imre Bodó, Lawrence Alderson and Bertrand Langlois

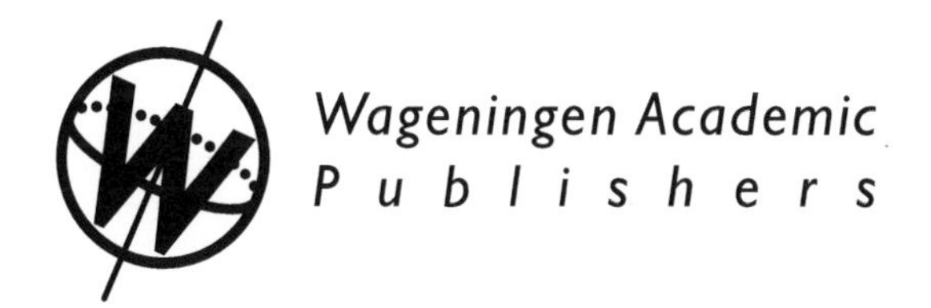

Subject headings:
Molecular methods
Use of markers
Genetic diversity

ISBN 9076998795
ISSN 0071-2477

First published, 2005

Wageningen Academic Publishers
The Netherlands, 2005

Foreword

Until recently, breeding of productive horses, namely sport horses and increasingly race horses which are directly profitable for horse industry, was mainly subjected to genetic research. Using the modern knowledge obtained through other livestock , breeding sport horses in particular has been extensively improved. The harmonisation of the methods and tools for breeding sport horses is now in progress at the EU level thanks to a strong effort of European countries in the scope of "Interstallion working group" placed under the umbrella of WBFSH-EAAP-ICAR. However, the horse industry could be faced in the future, as are other livestock industries, with the demand to preserve some genetic diversity as crossbreeding between European sport breeds increases.

Equids (horses and asses) have a particular place in the human culture and history. There are strong historical links between equids breeds and particular geographical or/and ecological areas. Equids contribute actively to the preservation of local or national history as they are as much a part of the patrimony as is historical architecture.

In Europe, agricultural policy is more and more focused on the concept of global management and on the promotion of sustainable agriculture. The so-called "second pillar" of the common agricultural policy aims to guarantee the future of rural areas including social and economics needs (European commission 2001). Production and utilisation of equids can play a significant role in this new challenge as evidenced at the symposium on Livestock Production Farming systems held in Benevento, Italy on 25/26 August 2003. (see report entitled *" Local animal resources and products in sustainable developement: role and potential of equids"*). The equids industry can fulfil this demand as the production and utilisation of equids are so diversified. Equids are bred for work, races, sports, hacking, forestry, agritourism, sociocultural events etc. Equids are involved in pastoral management providing output (work, meat, milk) from grassland and they contribute to the preservation of biodiversity and landscape. Equids contribute to maintain population in rural areas as they provide supplementary incomes and maintain traditional cultural events that highlight the rural scene. Equids are good mediators for citizens who are attempting to again join the rural way of life or/and to practice new sports in the periurban areas or/and in the countryside or in natural parks. Finally, equids federate a global approach in the valorisation of the patrimony. This evolution is supported by several European countries.

The preservation and exploitation of equids biodiversity is thus becoming an important issue in reference to the increase in intensive breeding of sport horses and to the socio-economics role and input of equids. Many equid breeds that occupy special niches and contribute to biodiversity safeguards, exist in European countries. Some populations, and namely rare breeds need to be re-evaluated yet, others need to be saved from extinction very quickly. Hence, it was the right time for Horse Commission to perform a session devoted to this topic at the 55th annual meeting of EAAP held in Bled, Slovenia. This session was prepared, carried out and is now published jointly by Horse commission of EAAP and Rare Breeds International (RBI) organisation.

RBI is active in working to conserve endangered equine breeds in many parts of the world. It acts as a focal point for the collation and dissemination of information and receives notification of threatened populations such as Abaco horses, Sardinian donkeys and Skyros ponies. It maintains an overview of local projects by national organisations to support native breeds, and assisted the successful efforts in Australia to conserve the Coffin Bay horses in their original location. Similarly, it made strong representations to maintain support for endangered equine breeds in the UK when proposed changes to the British Horserace Board threatened the security of several breeds. In various circumstances it acts directly when appropriate. For instance: a project to provide support for Turkoman horses in Iran was implemented with the aid of a grant from a charitable foundation in the USA. Funds were allocated for the purchase of animals, provision of feed and water, and to develop a system of recording and DNA profiling.

Its activities cover a comprehensive range of functions from political to cultural promotion. On one hand, it was represented on an Equine Breed Definition Working Group examining Commission Decision 92/353/EEC and Commission Decision 96/78/EEC. On the other hand, it organised an exhibition of bronze equine sculptures by the highly acclaimed sculptor, Nicola Toms, in London in support of endangered breeds.

There is a consensus among scientists and organisations that preservation of equids can be investigated using modern concepts, methods and tools of quantitative genetics and molecular biology . Such attempts have been very successful for Lippizan breeds in the late 20th century with the support of EAAP and European community (Copernicus project 1997-2000: final report INCO-COPERNICUS IC15CT96-0904). These results were presented in a session performed by Horse commission at the 52th annual meeting of EAAP held in Budapest, Hungary. In the meantime this kind of investigation is extended to other rare breeds by different European groups. This publication aims to provide a general overview of what research has been recently carried out, identifies the most relevant data, and makes similar attempts to identify research conducted regarding sport horses. Finally, there is a discussion of the prospect for a coordinated research effort at the EU level in the scope of an informal working group to be designed under the umbrella of EAAP and RBI.

Dr William Martin-Rosset
President of Horse commission at EAAP

Table of contents

Introduction

The conservation of the wealth of genetic diversity inherited from the past is becoming increasingly important for the quality of life of mankind, even though often it is not economic. For the future, however, it is a very important activity and the reasons for the maintenance of breeds of domestic animals - cattle, sheep, swine, poultry and horses - are based on both cultural and technical arguments.

The aspect of human culture relates not only to aesthetical, educational and historical aspects, but also to rural tourism, and the maintenance of the environment and regional character. At the same time, there are many technical arguments for the maintenance of genetic resources. They are an insurance against changing requirements for animal production in the future; marginal areas can be utilized by traditional livestock; maternal lines of rare breeds usually are productive in modern cross breeding systems; and the products of traditional local breeds provide quality for growing niche markets.

Despite these strong arguments for the maintenance of traditional native breeds, they do not always result in profitable business. Therefore conservation must be subsidised, but the sources of funds are limited and it is not possible to subsidise all endangered breed populations throughout the world.

Thus the prioritisation of support for rare breeds demands consideration of many factors. In some cases a small national population of a breed may be part of a larger global population which is not endangered. For example, in some countries a small population of Arabian horses or even English Thoroughbreds are on the list of endangered breeds, albeit they are not endangered international breeds. In other cases, such as the German Sporthorse breeds, a breed continues to exist with the same name but transformed for modern breeding goals by the introduction of foreign genes. Often there are different types within one breed (e.g. riding and driving Lipizzans), or the same type of animals may exist within different breeds (e.g. modern Sport horse type in Selle Français, Holstein, Hannover, Westfahlian, etc).

Therefore it is helpful to enlist the aid of modern science. The development of science, and molecular genetics in particular, already has given us many tools for reaching decisions to realise the preservation of different rare populations, whereas formerly it was necessary to rely solely on pedigree, conformation and historical data.

The various elements of a scientific approach - blood groups, polymorphisms, microsatellites and mitochondrial DNA - can show only a part of the genome. Molecular genetics assist conservation policy by relating geographical origin to the history and pedigree structure of a breed. They also enable analysis of reduced diversity in small populations. However, they are only element of a wider network of information, and the results of molecular genetics must be interpreted in the context of other evidence. *Cothran* noted that the scientifically based genetic distance can not be used alone to determine the uniqueness of the breed - „...the relation among breeds of species are more like a web than a tree".

Mitochondrial sequence data have clarified the nature of the domestication process in horses, pointing to a very restricted recruitment of males. Together with DNA sequence analyses, these methods have been used to define differences between breeds, to verify pedigree structures, to measure genetic variability in current populations and combimed with pedigree data, also in founder populations (*Cunningham*).

Molecular genetics can differentiate different groups of animals (*Ollivier et al.*), and it is possible to apply this approach to the classification of genetic diversity as proposed by J.J. Lauvergne (wild populations, primary traditional breeds, standardized breeds and selected lines).

It is important to review how genetic markers can help us to overcome difficulties resulting from reliance on pedigree information alone. The first result of immunogenetics, and later molecular genetics, was effective parentage verification by blood groups and other polymorphic systems. Now, improved DNA techniques, using about 20 polymorphic loci, have decreased incorrect exclusion to circa 0 %. Inbreeding is yet another field for the use of genetic markers.

Langlois shows, how genetic markers, if appropriately chosen like SNP, could improve the estimation of probability, that two alleles sorted at random in two individuals are identical by descent. Thus, it is possible to improve the parentage coefficient with the help of genetic markers when pedigree information is limited, which is mostly the case.

It is important and interesting to understand how the principles of conservation and the results of molecular genetics work in practice, and they are illustrated by the case studies described in this issue.

The Lipizzan is one of the most ancient breeds, having been established in 1580, and the stud books are more than two hundred year old. The mitochondrial study on this breed gives interesting results when compared with the data of pedigrees (*Dovć et al.*).

The Old Kladrub horse affords a good opportunity to study the genetic history of a two hundred years old breed, which suffered a serious bottleneck after World War II (*Jakubec et al.*).

L. Alderson gives us a comprehensive picture of native British horse and pony breeds, of which twelve endangered populations are listed in the Rare Breeds Survival Trust's categories. The evaluation was made on the basis of endangerment (population size) and between breeds diversity (genetic distance). Great Britain is interesting because it is the cradle of many founders and improvers of international horse breeds. The Irish Connemara breed (*Feely et al.*) belongs to the group of important rare breeds of Europe threatened by extinction by the increasing popularity of international riding pony.

The Bardigiano is a special Italian horse, which is selected increasingly for modern breeding objectives (*Fioretti et al.)*, while the paper by *Ivankovic et al.* showed that some native populations of horses in Croatia have been improved by crossing with other international breeds.

Hungary was famous for its horse breeding, and *Mihók et al.* compare two breeds which were established at an old State stud (Mezőhegyes, 1785) before they separated a half century later. Both were improved by English Thoroughbreds during the second half of the nineteenth century. Molecular genetics can provide evidence about the difference between these breeds, and reflect the influence of the English Thoroughbred

The Akhal Teke, alongside the Arabian, is another ancient distinct horse population. There are some individuals from this breed in different European countries but *A. Szontagh* studied it in its original country and hair samples were collected from the cradle of the breed in Turkmenistan.

Inbreeding always becomes a relevant factor when the traits of a new breed are being fixed (*Mantovani et al.*) and Northern Europe is the cradle of many breeds and valuable genes of horses. It is likely that one of the ancient ancestors of the species (Tarpan) is near to the horses of this region (*Saastamoinen et al.*). The paper by *Olsen et al* describes other northern breeds from Norway, such as the Døle and Nordland/Lyngen breeds, and the Zemaitukai horse, one of the famous and valuable horse breeds of Lithuania, is studied by *Juras and Cothran.*

Genetic characterisation and comparison of Pentro horses to Maremmano, Murgese, TPR, Haflinger, Standardbred and Bardigiano let us a look into the Spanish influence on horses in Italy (*Iamartino et al.*), and the paper by *Vega- Pla* details interesting histories of the introduction of different horse varieties to the American continent.

It is an excellent development, that so many data could be gathered from the genome of the horse. We have to consider, however, that this is only a small part of the genes and markers of the traits of the horse. Without doubt it will help to develop conservation policy, but **results of molecular genetics „...only in combination with all information about a rare breed can make a determination of whether the breed is worthy of conservation efforts"** (*Cothran*).

Molecular methods and equine genetic diversity

E.P. Cunningham

Trinity College Dublin, Ireland

Abstract

Since RFLPs became available in the 1980s, a sequence of developments (microsatellites, SNPs, sequencing) has greatly increased the power of molecular methods to describe, analyse and manage genetic variability. This paper reviews some results of these applications in horse populations. Mitochondrial sequence data have clarified the nature of the domestication process in horses, and show a pattern different from that in other domesticated species. Recent results point to a very restricted recruitment of males in the domestication process. Microsatellite (and increasingly SNP) data have clarified relationships between breeds worldwide. Deep pedigree structures have been studied closely in some populations (Lippizaner, Thoroughbred) using molecular methods. Finally, a new method, in which pedigree structures and molecular data are combined to give an estimate of genetic variability in founder populations, is presented.

Introduction

Prior to the development of methods for measuring genetic diversity at the DNA level in the 1980s, the possibilities for analysing the genetic structure or history of any species were quite limited. Despite this, the application of quantitative genetic analyses to phenotypic data, combined with analyses of population structures using pedigree data, had provided considerable insight into equine genetics. Heritabilities and genetic correlations for important traits were established, inbreeding patterns and their consequences were investigated, and patterns of inheritance of specific traits were clarified (Bowling and Ruvinsky, 2000).

Starting with the introduction of restriction fragment length polymorphisms (RFLPs) in 1980s a range of molecular techniques became available (Jeffreys *et al.*, 1987). These included the measurement of DNA sequences, the discovery of microsatellite diversity and a progressive increase in the power, speed and refinement of the methodologies involved. Application to mitochondrial and Y chromosome variation permitted the study of female and male genetic lineages.

Our work in applying quantitative genetic methodologies to horse populations began with early estimation of the inheritance of track performance (More O'Ferrall and Cunningham, 1974; Field and Cunningham, 1976), analyses of inbreeding and population structure (Mahon and Cunningham, 1982), and estimation of genetic trend in thoroughbred populations (Gaffney and Cunningham, 1988). As the molecular methods became available in the late 1980s, we began to apply them also to horse populations, with particular interest in the Thoroughbred. This paper reports on the results of that second cycle of molecular genetic studies in horses.

Molecular evidence of domestication

Because they are transmitted only through the female line, and are therefore not subject to recombination, mitochondrial DNA patterns are particularly useful for investigating the deep evolutionary background of any species. We have analysed mitochondrial variation in a wide range of horse populations and used the results to shed some light on the process of domestication in the horse (Hill *et al.*, 2002). Mitochondrial DNA sequences were determined by direct sequencing or inferred by comparative single strand conformation polymorphism (SSCP) analysis for 100 Thoroughbreds (blood samples). Further sequences were generated in the same way for 81 individuals (hair samples) from seven other horse populations [Far East: Tuva (n =11); Near East: Anatolian(n =13), Cukorova (n =12), Egyptian (n = 8), Fulani (n = 11); Europe: Connemara (n = 12), Shetland (n = 14)]. A further 28 sequences from six additional populations [Far East: Mongolian(n = 4), Cheju (n = 7), Tsushima (n = 2), Yunnan(n =2); Europe: Lippizan (n= 10), Belgian (n= 3)] were taken from GenBank. Complete data for all 14 populations were analysed for a 343bp sequence.

A total of 88 polymorphic sites (24 indels, 56 transitions, eight transversions) were found in this 343 bp fragment. These defined 92 sequences in the Thoroughbred and among the 109 individuals from the other 13 other geographically diverse populations. A total of 64 polymorphic sites defined 74 distinct haplotypes. Using these haplotypes, the phylogenetic relationships between the 13 modern horse populations and Thoroughbred founders were reconstructed in a neighbour-joining phylogeny (Figure 1). The labelled clades in this unrooted tree corresponded to those determined by Vila *et al.* (2001) although within this sequence no distinction was made between clades A and E.

No clear geographic affiliation of clades was apparent except clade F, which almost exclusively contained sequences from the Far East (frequency: 0.54) and the Near East (0.46) with the exception of one European (0.08) haplotype. No thoroughbred sequences were found within this clade.

The mean number of pairwise differences observed among all horse sequences was estimated as 7.51 or 2.30%. If the average rate of equid mtDNA divergence is assumed between 4.1 and 8.1% per million years (Vila *et al.*, 2001) then the average coalescence for modern horse mtDNA sequences is estimated between 280 000 (lower limit) and 560 000 (upper limit) years before present (YBP). This ancient divergence of horse lineages is supported in an analysis of population structure. When populations were grouped according to geographical origin (Far East: Cheju, Mongolian, Tsushima, Tuva, Yunnan; Near East: Anatolian, Cukorova, Egyptian, Fulani; Europe: Belgian, Connemara, Lippizan, Shetland), the greatest partitioning of genetic variation was detected among individuals within populations (92.4%). Although a significant proportion of the variation (7.9%) is partitioned non-randomly among regional populations, no difference was detected among the three regionally distinct groups, despite a tentative eastern-specific clade in the phylogeny. No indication of regional clustering of variation was detected from pairwise F_{ST} genetic distances between populations.

No difference in nucleotide diversity was detected between the Thoroughbred founders and contemporary horse populations. Sequence divergence ranged from 1.81% in the Fulani to 3.10% in the Tuva. Mean sequence diversity in the thoroughbred founder population (2.25%) was similar to estimates for the Anatolian (2.09%), Cheju (2.22%), Connemara (2.24%) and Cukorova (2.43%) populations.

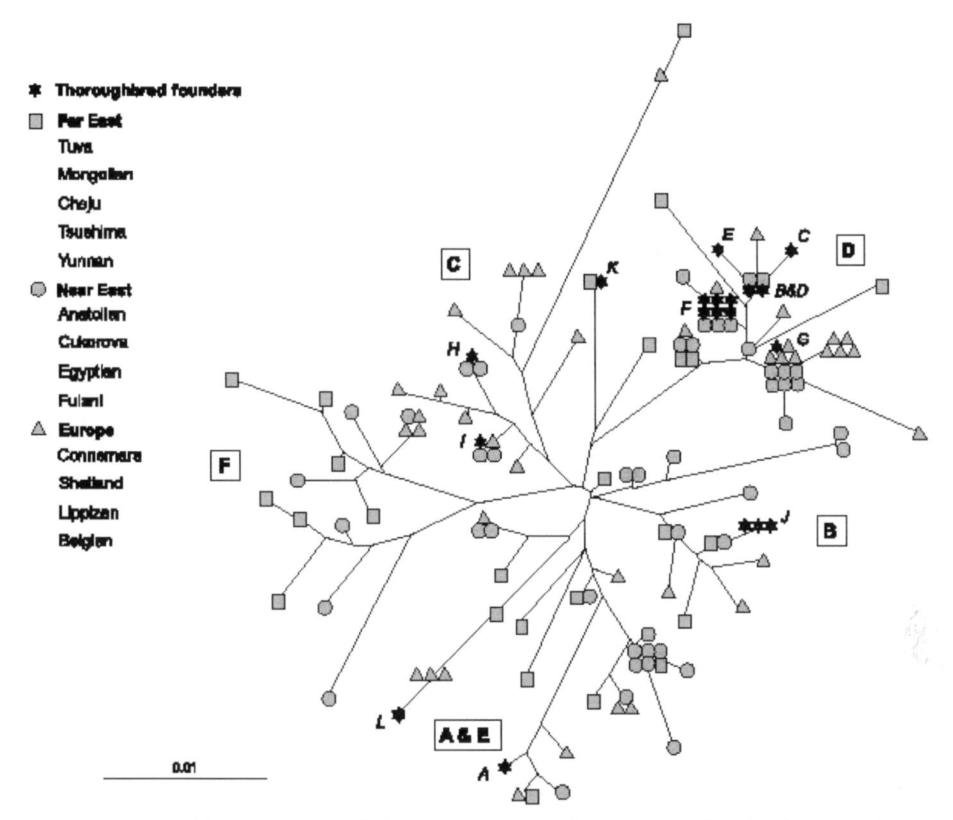

Figure 1. Neighbour-joining phylogenetic tree relating mitochondrial DNA (mtDNA) haplotypes in horse populations from three geographically widespread regions. A founder population for the thoroughbred was reconstructed from sequence and pedigree information and the haplotypes therein are represented in the tree as stars (Haplotypes A–L). Although considered separate founders in 381 bp Families 10 and 14 (Haplotypes B and D) share an identical sequence in 343 bp and therefore share the same node in this tree. Haplotypes cluster in five distinct clades similar to those determined by Vila et al. *(2001), although in this sequence, clades A and E are indistinguishable. Source: Hill* et al.*, 2002.*

These results are broadly in line with those from two other studies; (Vila *et al.,* 2001) and (Jansen *et al.,* 2002). They indicate a pattern of domestication in the horse which is quite different to that inferred for other species. Loftus *et al.* (1994) were the first to demonstrate, using mitochondrial data, a clear dual domestication of cattle. Their evidence showed that the mitochondrial divergence between cattle from the Indian subcontinent on the one hand and those from Africa and Europe on the other was so deep rooted that they could not have been domesticated from a common population of wild ancestors. Similar results have since been demonstrated in goats, sheep, swine and water buffalo. In contrast, the results from horses show no such clear distinctions that can be linked to geographical origins. This suggests that though the domestication process may well have taken in mitochondrial variants from across the full range of the wild species, there has been so much interchange of genetic material between populations in the 6,000+ years since domestication that the results of any such wide sampling are now spread throughout today's breeds.

Recent work (Lindgren *et al.*, 2004) on Y chromosome variation has shown a totally contrasting picture for male transmitted DNA. Among twenty two separate populations, they found only a single pattern of Y chromosome.

Origins of the Thoroughbred – pedigree analyses

Relationships between individuals can be measured in terms of the probability that they share ancestral genetic material. This concept, now known as identity by descent (IBD) was developed by Wright (1922) and Malecot (1948) to construct methods by which relationships can be calculated if pedigree structure is known. Malecot's *Coefficient de Parenté* (in English, the co-ancestry coefficient or CC) is now the standard measure of genetic relationship.

In the case of the Thoroughbred, recorded pedigrees go back more than three hundred years, and more than thirty generations. Towards the end of the 17th Century, significant numbers of horses with Arabian, Turk and Barb ancestry were imported into Britain (Willett, 1975). In 1791, a general studbook (GSB) was established by James Weatherby, and from that date virtually all thoroughbreds are descended from animals already registered.

In an early study (Mahon and Cunningham, 1982) we used these pedigree records to estimate recent and long term inbreeding in the population, and to calculate its relationship to fertility. In a more recent study (Cunningham *et al.*, 2001) we have used the complete archive of pedigree records for the thoroughbred (approximately one million horses) to examine the impact of founder animals on the structure of the population.

The CC between a founder and a later-born animal is a measure of the genetic contribution of that foundation animal to the latter-day individual. The genetic contribution of each foundation animal was investigated in samples of 200 horses born in 20-year intervals from 1770 to 1990. Founder horses were defined as those born prior to 1750 which had two unknown parents. If a horse had only one parent unknown, the unknown parent was considered a founder animal.

The total number of founders identified was 158, of which 85 were male. Their contributions to the current population are very unequal, varying downwards from a maximum of 13.53% (Godolphin Arabian). These contributions were used to calculate the effective number of founders Nef = 28.15. This is the theoretical number of equally contributing founders which would be expected to produce the same genetic diversity as found in the current population.

All horses in the dataset were traced through their paternal lineages until a male with unknown sire was found. In total, 85 such terminal foundation sires, born from 1665 to 1860, were identified. Percentage contributions of leading foundation sires were examined for each decade from 1725 to 1995. In a similar analysis, all horses in the dataset were traced along their maternal lineages until a terminal dam was found, and the contributions of the female founders were calculated.

Not all founders contributed equally to subsequent generations. The 10 founders with the highest contribution were responsible for 45% of genetic makeup in the 1990 sample. The top 20 founders contributed 65% of genes and the top 30 founders 78%. The contribution of all 158 identified founders amounted to 81%. The most significant founders were the Godolphin Arabian (13.8%), the Darley Arabian (6.5%), the Curwen Bay Barb (4.2%), the Ruby Mare

(4.2%) and the Byerley Turk (3.3%). The total and relative contributions of the top 10 founders were practically identical in each cohort since 1790. This confirms the conclusion (McPhee and Wright, 1925; Gandini *et al.,* 1997) that relative founder contributions become established very early in closed populations and are subsequently very stable. It is also consistent with the demonstration (Caballero and Toro, 2000) that Nef, the effective number of founders, becomes a constant after a short number of generations.

While other stallions were responsible for paternal lineages early in the history of Thoroughbreds, by the mid-1800s only three remained: the Byerley Turk, the Darley Arabian and the Godolphin Arabian. The percentage of paternal lineages attributable to the Darley Arabian line has been increasing for nearly 175 years, and is now responsible for 95% of paternal lineages in the modern population. Each of these three foundation stallions is linked to the population in paternal lineage through contributions of only one of their male-line descendants. The influence of the Byerley Turk is carried on through his great great grandson Herod (1758), the Darley Arabian through his great great grandson Eclipse (1764) and the Godolphin Arabian through his grandson Matchem (1748).

The 10 foundation dams with the greatest contribution to horses born from 1985 to 1994 accounted for 72% of maternal lineages. The top 20 founder females were responsible for 89% of maternal lineages in this decade, while the top 30 accounted for 94% of maternal lineages. A study (Bowling *et al.,* 2000) of American-born Arabian horses has produced similar results, indicating that 28 maternal lineages account for greater than 89% of the modern population.

Molecular measurement of Thoroughbred maternal lineages

A system for the classification of thoroughbred female lines was devised by the end of the 19th century that traced all mares in the GSB at that time as far back as possible in direct maternal descent to one of 43 founder mares, descendants of which are considered a family. These are ranked in order of the number of Classic race winners prior to 1890 that were members of that family and named according to that rank, i.e. Family 1 had the most Classic race winners, Family 2 the second most, etc. (Lowe, 1913). Today, family assignment is often considered an important indicator of genetic value within the Thoroughbred industry. Also, specific mating combinations between families are sometimes considered more or less auspicious than others. We have used this system to identify descendants of 19 of the most common female families (Table 1) in a large resource of thoroughbreds.

Mitochondrial DNA (mtDNA) haplotypes should be shared by all individuals within a family. Stability of maternal inheritance within documented horse pedigrees has been demonstrated in both Lippizan (> 200 years) (Kavar *et al.,* 1999) and Arabian (100 years) (Bowling *et al.,* 2000) horses.

Mitochondrial DNA sequences were determined by direct sequencing or inferred by comparative single strand conformation polymorphism (SSCP) analysis for 100 thoroughbreds (blood samples) representing 19 female families A total of 39 polymorphic sites (three indels, 35 transitions, one transversion) were found in a 381 bp mtDNA D-loop fragment.When insertion/deletion events were ignored, 17 haplotypes were found to have contributed to the 19 female lineages. However, only 11 families conserved a single haplotype, i.e. more than one haplotype was detected within eight of the 19 families (Table 1). In six of these eight mismatched families there was one predominant sequence with a single mismatched sample. Anomalous sequences in two families (Families 11 and 12) differed from the numerically predominant (majority) sequence in the family by only one nucleotide substitution and it is possible that these two could be a result of *de novo* mutation.

Table 1. Thoroughbred founder females considered by historical pedigree records and by genetics illustrating the extent of sequence sharing among families and the occurrence of anomalous sequences within families. In families with more than one sequence, the founder haplotype is indicated by an asterisk. Source: Hill et al., *2002.*

Family no.	Founder mare	Approximate date	*n*	Haplotypes	Type of anomaly
1	Tregonwell's Natural Barb Mare	1657-1670	9	F, H*	MOD
2	Burton's Barb Mare	1660-1685	7	F	-
3	Dam of the Two True Blues	1690	6	E	-
4	Layton Barb Mare	1650	10	J	-
5	Massey Mare	1714	4	L*, M	DR
6	Old Morocco Mare	1656	3	C*, N	DR
7	Lord Darcy's Blacklegged Royal Mare	1710	5	F	-
8	Bustler Mare	1680	6	F	-
9	Old Spot Mare	1700	10	A*, G	DR
10	Grey Childers Mare	1741	1	B	-
11	The Pet Mare	1697	4	J*, L, P	MOD & MUT
12	Royal Mare	1700	3	G*, Q	MUT
13	Sedbury Royal Mare	1665	6	J	-
14	Oldfield Mare	1695	7	D	-
16	Hutton's Old Spot Mare	1695	8	F*, H	MOD
17	Byerley Turk Mare	1700-1710	2	F	-
19	Davill's Woodcock Mare	1690	7	K*, O	MOD
22	Belgrade Turk Mare	1718	1	F	-
25	Brimmer Mare	1699	1	I	-

MOD: Relatively recent anomaly in modern pedigree; DR: deep rooted anomaly, possible foundation stage confusion; MUT: possible *de novo* mutation; *Founder haplotype.

We suggest that the extent of nucleotide differences (>2–14 nt) between the majority and anomalous sequences in the other heterogenous families (Families 1, 5, 6, 9, 11, 16 and 19) are best explained by confusion between horses from either another family sharing the anomalous sequence, a family not represented in this sample, or a non-thoroughbred. One family (Family 11) had two aberrant sequences and in another family (Family 9) two sequences were represented approximately equally (11 nt divergent). Pedigree analysis has allowed some determination of the anomalies in time, indicating some possible foundation stage confusions where these occur at a potentially deep root in a pedigree

In order to reconstruct a founder population (1650– 1750 AD) for the Thoroughbred we assumed that the majority haplotype within each maternal lineage family represented the founder sequence. In Family 9, two sequences were detected in approximately equal proportions. One of them the was not shared with any other family (A), and this was taken as the founder haplotype. Following this assumption, we have identified 12 distinct founder haplotypes (A–L). Ten of these founder haplotypes (A–E, G–I, K–L) were unique to single families and two (F, J) were shared by more than one family. The remaining five haplotypes may have arisen by mutation or derive from a family founder not represented in this study (M–Q)

The examination of detailed pedigree records documenting the history of the Thoroughbred, coupled with mtDNA sequence analysis, has facilitated this first in-depth investigation of the founder mares. Genetic diversity estimates in the thoroughbred female founders are not dissimilar to observed estimates in contemporary horse populations. However, the examination of horse population diversity reveals a consistent absence of geographical structure and a lack of phylogenetic sorting of haplotypes into divergent but inwardly invariant groups as seen in other large domesticates (MacHugh and Bradley, 2001). Such heterogenous genetic origins of the horse prevent us from making any firm statement about Thoroughbred origins per se – Thoroughbreds might equally descend from a single diverse source population as they may have evolved from several populations, though historical records suggest the latter (Willett, 1975). The uncertainty of the genetic origins of the thoroughbred is a consequence of the domestication history of the horse. High diversity estimates, limited definitive haplotype clustering within populations and random distribution of diversity among horse populations is consistent with the capture and exploitation of genetically diverse wild progenitors having taken place in multiple locations, possibly over a broad time span throughout the >6000 years association between humans and the horse (Vila *et al.,* 2001). The high mobility of the horse, enabled by the nature of its domestic roles will also have led to an obscuring of the genetic structure within the species through post-domestic migration.

Haplotype sharing among thoroughbred founders is much higher than observed in other horse populations. The estimated PI in the thoroughbred founder population (0.15) suggests that at least 15 in 100 randomly sampled thoroughbreds (given that all founder lineages are represented equally) share an identical sequence. This is three times the observed PI in Arabian horses (0.05) (Bowling et al. 2000) and higher than in all other populations examined here except the Fulani (0.24) and Shetland (0.23), though these estimates may be biased by unintentional sampling of relatives. In the thoroughbred, because PI estimates are much higher in founders than expected we propose that some thoroughbred lineages may descend from common dams. For example, the coupling of this genetic information with pedigree records strongly indicates that Families 4 (Layton Barb Mare 1670), 11 (The Pet Mare 1697) and 13 (Sedbury Royal Mare 1665) may descend from a single common founder. The founder haplotype in each is identical (Haplotype J), all three were owned by James Darcy, were kept at Sedbury Stud and lived at about the same time.

We propose that as few as 12 founders may have contributed to the major lineages within the 19 thoroughbred families included in this study. However, if we also consider the deep-rooted anomalies, which probably result from confusion at the foundation stages, then Families 5 and 6 both have a contribution from an additional founder (Haplotypes M and N). The deep-rooted Family 9 anomaly (Hapolype G) may best be explained by confusion with the founder of Family 12. In fact, only one anomalous haplotype (Haplotype O, Family 19) in a relatively modern pedigree (19th century – 1980) is not accounted for by a match with another sampled family.

Although each family is expected to have only one founder and this founder is considered to contribute to one family only we have uncovered a web of founder sharing. Female founders, as they are currently understood, may have contributed differently to these 19 families than previously thought. Further, descendants of Maid of the Glen 1858 (1), Hag 1744 (5), the dam(s) of Betty Percival 1715 and Cream Cheeks 1695 (6), a Curwen Bay Barb Mare 1708/1709 (9), Young Camilla 1787 (11), Lady Alice 1855 (16) and Violet 1858 (19) (Fig. 1) may contain a genetic heritage different to that which pedigree information suggests.

The coupling of genetic and historical data provides a powerful tool to identify and correct errors that may be present in contemporary thoroughbred pedigrees. This is vital for thoroughbred breeders who rely on the accuracy of stud books, as important breeding decisions are frequently made based on the integrity of the pedigrees. Also, such parallel analyses lend new perspective to the interpretation of the early history of the thoroughbred and the contribution of the founder mares to the present day thoroughbred gene pool.

Comparative microsatellite analysis of Thoroughbred genetic diversity

The average proportion of allele sharing (APS) among individuals within and between each of four breed groups is shown in Table 2. The expected and observed heterozygosities are also given for each population, together with the allelic diversity, measured as the average number of alleles per locus. Both Shetland (SH) and Thoroughbred showed departure from Hardy-Weinberg equilibrium ($P < 0.01$) at three loci whilst the Egyptian and Turkish samples showing departure are one locus each.

Table 2. Comparison of thoroughbred, Shetland, Egyptian and Turkish horses at 13 microsatellite loci. Source: Cunningham et al.*, 2001.*

Population	*n*	Average no. of alleles/loci[1]	Heterozygosity		APS[2]			
			Observed	Expected	TB	SH	EG	TU
Thoroughbred (TB)	211	4.7 (4.3)	0.628	0.646	0.469	0.269	0.354	0.335
Shetland (SH)	40	5.3 (5.2)	0.642	0.661		0.449	0.276	0.290
Egyptian (EG)	34	6.0 (6.0)	0.654	0.691			0.396	0.365
Turkish (TU)	43	7.5 (7.4)	0.671	0.732				0.356

[1]Figures in parentheses are values at equal sample size of 34.
[2]Average proportion of alleles shared.

The level of allele sharing (APS) within a population is one indicator of genetic diversity. The lower the APS, the greater the diversity. With an APS of 0.469, the TB showed significantly less diversity that EG and TU, with APS of 0.396 and 0.356, respectively. The SH had a high level of allele sharing, similar to that in TB, reflecting the effectively closed nature of these two populations. The APS within each population was less than would be expected under random breeding (by 1.3, 1.5, 5.7 and 7.4% in TB, SH, EG and TU, respectively), reflecting breeding practices which avoid mating close relatives. Table 1 shows a consistent level of allele sharing within and between EG and TU, and between them and TB. Because many of the early individuals instrumental in the formation of TB were imported from the Middle East (Willet, 1975), this result is not surprising. In contrast, the lower level of allele sharing of all three with SH confirms the different background of that breed. Further evidence of breed relationships is given by the particular alleles which breeds have in common. Of 61 total alleles in TB, 10 were not found in SH but only two were absent from either EG or TU. A useful measure of genetic diversity, sometimes called 'allelic diversity' is given by the average number of alleles per locus in a population. Thoroughbreds had 37% fewer alleles than EG or TU, the difference being the result of the least frequent alleles in EG or TU being absent from TB.

Measuring genetic diversity in Thoroughbred founders by combined use of population and molecular methods

The regression of APS on CC was calculated. It gave an intercept of 0.309 and a regression of 1.013 (Figure 2). The almost perfect linear relationship confirms that these two measures of genetic relationship are in fact measuring the same thing. Because Thoroughbreds have been an effectively closed population for a large number of generations, no animal pair in today's population would be found to have a CC of zero. However, CC is calculated relative to some base group beyond which no further pedigree information is available and whose members are assumed to be unrelated and therefore to have an average CC of zero. The intercept, 0.309, is the estimated APS among these founder animals. This combination of molecular and statistical measures of relationships therefore provides a way of estimating genetic variability in founder groups. The founders of the Thoroughbred, with APS of 0.309 seem to have been more genetically diverse than present day Turkish and Egyptian populations with APS of 0.396 and 0.356, respectively.

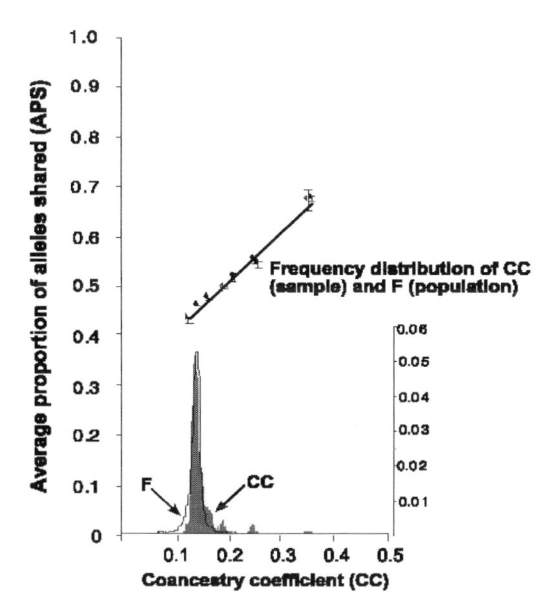

Figure 2. The relationship between molecular (average proportion of alleles shared, APS) and statistical (coeffcient of coancestry, CC) measures of alleles shared between all pairs of individuals in a sample of 211 thoroughbred (TB) horses. The CC values were grouped in 0·05 intervals and mean APS and CC values were calculated for each interval. The frequency distribution of CC values for all pairs of individuals in the sample is shown (right hand scale). The regression of APS on CC was close to unity at 1.013, indicating that molecular measures can concern average allele sharing calculated from pedigrees. The intercept (0.309) allows an estimated proportion of allele sharing among the founders of the thoroughbred population at about 31%. Source: Cunningham et al., *2001.*

References

Bowling, A.T., A. Del Valle and M. Bowling, 2000. A pedigree-based study of mitochondrial D-loop DNA sequence variation among Arabian horses. Anim Genet 31: 1-7.

Bowling, A.T. and A. Ruvinsky, 2000. Genetics of the Horse. CABI publishing.

Caballero, A. and M.A. Toro, 2000. Interrelations between effective population size and other pedigree tools for the management of conserved populations. Genet Res 75: 331-343.

Cunningham, E.P., J.J. Dooley, R.K. Splan and D.G. Bradley, 2001. Microsatellite diversity, pedigree relatedness and the contributions of founder lineages to thoroughbred horses. Anim Genet 32: 360-364.

Field, J.K. and E.P. Cunningham, 1976. A further study of the inheritance of racing performance in thoroughbred horses. J Hered 67: 247-248.

Gaffney, B. and E.P. Cunningham, 1988. Estimation of genetic trend in racing performance of thoroughbred horses. Nature 332: 722-724.

Gandini, G.C., A. Samore and G. Pagnacco, 1997. Genetic contribution of the Arabian to the Italian HaØinger horse. Journal of Animal Breeding and Genetics 114: 457-464.

Hill, E.W., D.G. Bradley, M. Al-Barody, O. Ertugrul, R.K. Splan, I. Zakharov and E.P. Cunningham, 2002. History and integrity of thoroughbred dam lines revealed in equine mtDNA variation. Anim Genet 33: 287-294.

Jansen, T., P. Forster, M.A. Levine, H. Oelke, M. Hurles, C. Renfrew, J. Weber and K. Olek, 2002. Mitochondrial DNA and the origins of the domestic horse. Proc Natl Acad Sci U S A 99: 10905-10910.

Jeffreys, A.J., V. Wilson, Z. Wong, N. Royle, I. Patel, R. Kelly and R. Clarkson, 1987. Highly variable minisatellites and DNA fingerprints. Biochem Soc Symp 53: 165-180.

Kavar, T., F. Habe, G. Brem and P. Dovc, 1999. Mitochondrial D-loop sequence variation among the 16 maternal lines of the Lipizzan horse breed. Anim Genet 30: 423-430.

Lindgren, G., N. Backstrom, J. Swinburne, L. Hellborg, A. Einarsson, K. Sandberg, G. Cothran, C. Vila, M. Binns and H. Ellegren, 2004. Limited number of patrilines in horse domestication. Nat Genet 36: 335-336.

Loftus, R.T., D.E. Machugh, D.G. Bradley, P.M. Sharp and P. Cunningham, 1994. Evidence for two independent domestications of cattle. Proc Natl Acad Sci U S A 91: 2757-2761.

Lowe, C.B., 1913. Breeding racehorses by the figure system. In: The Field and Queen, edited by W. Allison. (Horace Cox) Ltd, UK.

MacHugh, D.E. and D.G. Bradley, 2001. Livestock genetic origins: goats buck the trend. Proc Natl Acad Sci U S A 98: 5382-5384.

Mahon, G.A.T. and E.P. Cunningham, 1982. Inbreeding and the inheritance of fertility in the thoroughbred mare. Livestock Production Science 9: 743-754.

Malécot, G., 1948. Les mathématiques de l'hérédité. Masson, Paris.

McPhee, H.C. and S. Wright, 1925. Mendelian analysis of the pure breeds of livestock. III. The Shorthorns. Journal of Heredity 16: 205-215.

More O'Ferrall, G.J. and E.P. Cunningham, 1974. Heritability of racing performance in thoroughbred horses. Livestock Production Science 1: 87-97.

Vila, C., J.A. Leonard, A. Gotherstrom, S. Marklund, K. Sandberg, K. Liden, R.K. Wayne and H. Ellegren, 2001. Widespread origins of domestic horse lineages. Science 291: 474-477.

Willett, P., 1975. An Introduction to the Thoroughbred. Stanley Paul Ltd., London.

Wright, S., 1922. Coefficients of inbreeding and relationship. American Naturalist 56: 330-338.

The use of markers for characterising genetic resources[1]

L. Ollivier[1], C. Chevalet[2] and J.L. Foulley[1]

[1]INRA, Station de Génétique Quantitative et Appliquée, 78352 Jouy-en-Josas cedex, France
[2]INRA, Laboratoire de Génétique Cellulaire, BP 27, 31326 Castanet-Tolosan cedex, France

Abstract

Methods for characterising genetic resources on the basis of molecular markers are reviewed. Genetic variability between breeds is generally based on a set of allelic frequencies. Usual expressions of diversity are fixation (or gene diversity) indices proposed by Wright (or Nei), and pair wise genetic distances between breeds. Genetic distances may be used to build phylogenetic trees, to perform breed clustering, or to derive global measures of diversity. Allelic richness brings useful complementary information. Experimental designs for diversity studies and statistical reliability are briefly discussed.

Keywords: marker, genetic diversity, allelic richness, genetic distance

Introduction

As underlined in the French chart for the management of genetic resources (BRG, 1999), the better the available genetic resources are characterised the better they can be used. Several levels of characterisation exist. First, breed inventories are being made to collect information aiming at a wide coverage of the populations making the genetic resources of each species. This kind of information is nowadays stored in databases, either at country, European or global level. Let us recall that those resources may be classified according to an evolutionary scale, as proposed by Lauvergne (1982). Four categories of populations may be distinguished, namely wild populations, primary (or traditional) populations, standardised breeds and selected lines. Those categories reflect different domestication status and successive steps in the general domestication process. Breed inventories, however, apart from some succinct information on the production characteristics of the various breeds, do not tell us much about their resemblances or dissimilarities, and thus on their diversity. Genetic markers offer the great advantage of a direct assessment of genetic diversity, by definition independent from environmental effects. The question is of course to know whether the markers variability well reflects variability at quantitative trait loci, for instance variability of production or adaptation traits. This aspect, out of the scope of the present article, has been discussed by Barker (2001) who reports on several studies of natural populations and plants showing that the two variabilities are often connected, even though the degree of those connexions and their generality remain a matter of debate.

Molecular markers have a set of properties that make them a tool of choice in the evaluation of genetic variability within-breed as well as between-breed. Let us mention their polymorphism, their ubiquity over the genome and the possibility of automating their identification. Other genetic markers, which have been used to characterise diversity for more

[1]Translated from: Ollivier, L., Chevalet C. and J.-L. Foulley, 2000. Utilisation des marqueurs pour la caractérisation des ressources génétiques. INRA Productions Animales, 2000, no hors série « Génétique moléculaire : principes et applications aux populations animales », 247-252.

than 40 years, do not generally cumulate the advantages mentioned above. On this aspect one may consult, among many others, two studies on French cattle breeds by Grosclaude *et al.* (1990) and Moazami-Goudarzi *et al.* (1997), based on biochemical and molecular markers respectively. We intend here to provide an overview of the methods of characterisation based on molecular markers, for which an increasing amount of data becomes now available in all farm animal species.

Fixation indices of Wright and gene diversity of Nei

The most classical method for characterising populations' diversity, and perhaps also the earliest, is the use of *fixation indices* (F) proposed by Wright in 1943 (cited by Nei, 1977), who defines three F coefficients related as follows:

$$(1 - F_{IT}) = (1 - F_{IS})(1 - F_{ST}) \quad (1)$$

These Fs generalise the coefficient of inbreeding by extending it to the case of subdivided populations. F_{IT} is the inbreeding (or correlation between uniting gametes in Wright's terminology) of *individuals* in the *total* population (IT), whereas F_{IS} is the inbreeding of *individuals* in each *sub-population* (IS). F_{ST} is not properly speaking a fixation index, since it designates the correlation between two gametes taken at random in two *sub-populations* from the *total* population (ST). F_{ST} measures the degree of genetic differentiation of the sub-populations. Those Fs may also be defined in the probabilistic approach of Malécot (though F_{IS} and F_{IT} may take negative values). It is to be noted that they are statistical parameters (correlations or probabilities) requiring only pedigrees and no real genotypes.

A different approach has been proposed by Nei (1973), based on actual heterozygosities (H) at several loci. Nei defines a concept of *gene diversity* and shows that total gene diversity (H_T) can be partitioned into intrasubpopulational (H_S) and intersubpopulational (D_{ST}) gene diversities, so that $H_T = H_S + D_{ST}$. The heterozygosities H_T and H_S are those expected under the hypothesis of Hardy-Weinberg equilibrium and therefore only depend on the observed allelic frequencies. Nei then defines F indices similar to those of Wright, from the *expected* heterozygosities (H_T and H_S) and the *observed* total heterozygosity (H_O), averaged over several loci, as follows:

$$F_{IT} = 1 - H_O / H_T, \; F_{IS} = 1 - H_O / H_S \text{ et } F_{ST} = 1 - H_S / H_T \quad (2)$$

One can see that the Fs so defined also satisfy equation (1). Nei also defines a *coefficient of gene differentiation* (G_{ST}) such that $G_{ST} = D_{ST}/H_T$. This G_{ST} is similar in form to - though different from – the F_{ST} of Wright. Conceptually, Wright considers the situation of one locus over a large number of populations, whereas Nei considers the inverse situation of several loci – with the aim of evaluating the genome diversity – over a limited number of real populations.

Genetic distance, phylogeny and diversity

Gene differentiation, as expressed by the G_{ST} of Nei defined above, also applies to the extreme case of two sub-populations, and it can then be considered as a measure of the *genetic distance* between them. One of the first measures of distance proposed has indeed been the F_{ST} distance of Latter (1972), also akin to the distance of Reynolds (see the Appendix for the definition of those distances). Since G_{ST}, from the definition given above, is a function only of heterozygosities H_T and H_S under Hardy-Weinberg equilibrium, this distance is a function only of the gene frequencies in the two sub-populations. Several other measures of distance have been proposed (see Nei, 1987). They all similarly depend only on the gene frequencies (these are called x_{ij} and y_{ij} in the Appendix summarising the most used distances). In passing we may note that distances between individuals may also be calculated on the basis of their genotypes, by using a multi-locus estimation of kinship (as proposed, for instance, by Chevalet, 1980).

When a set of N sub-populations is available, a matrix (N × N) of pair wise distances can be established. Such a matrix allows deriving a *phylogeny*, based on the idea that the genetic distance separating two sub-populations is proportional to the time elapsed since they diverged from a common sub-population-ancestor. When distances are based on variation of DNA sequence – as mainly in studies of interspecific diversity – the basic hypothesis is the constancy of sequence's evolution, the so-called "molecular clock". In the case of allelic frequency, which is of interest here, divergence is supposed to be the result of a genetic drift process, and the corresponding hypothesis therefore is the uniform pace of genetic drift, which implies sub-populations of uniform effective size. The algorithms for phylogenetic tree reconstruction from a distance matrix, and the way to calculate the branch lengths are described in detail by Hartl and Clark (1997, p. 368-372).

The number of possible trees, or topologies, increases rapidly with N, since for N=10 sub-populations the number of trees possible *a priori* already exceeds 34×10^6. The topology obtained from a set of distances is in fact the most likely one in a vast number of possibilities. The question of its degree of reliability is then raised. Reliability is usually assessed via the "bootstrap[2]" technique. The idea is to re-sample the original data, by randomly drawing with replacement a sample of the 2n alleles present at each locus in the original sample of n individuals, or by similarly drawing the L loci sampled. The frequency of occurrence of each node of the initial tree on a large number of re-samplings (e. g. 1000) is then taken as a reliability criterion (Felsenstein, 1985). A significance threshold may be retained, for instance 5% if the node occurs in 95% of the samples. We may note that the statistical validity of this technique rests on the strong hypothesis of homogeneity of the experimental units, which may not be verified in particular for different loci. An example of phylogenetic tree, constructed from distances among French breeds of cattle (Moazami-Goudarzi *et al.*, 1997), is given in Figure 1. One can see that this tree is not very reliable, since no node reaches the 5 % threshold.

The genetic distances matrix may also serve to evaluate the *global diversity* of a set S of breeds, using the approach advocated by Weitzman (1993). He defines a diversity function V(S), which is the maximum, over all breeds of the set S, of the distance (d_i) between breed i and the closest breed in set S, plus the diversity of the subset S_i obtained by excluding breed i, and is written:

$$V(S) = \text{maximum over S of } [d_i + V(S_i)] \qquad (3)$$

[2] According to Robert (1992), the word bootstrap alludes to a story told by Cyrano de Bergerac (*Histoire Comique Contenant les Essais et Empires de la Lune*, 1657), in which the main character reaches the moon by drawing on his "bootstraps". But the inventor of the bootstrap technique appears to have himself been ignorant of Cyrano and was making reference to a similar story told by a German writer of the 18th century (D. Laloë, personal communication).

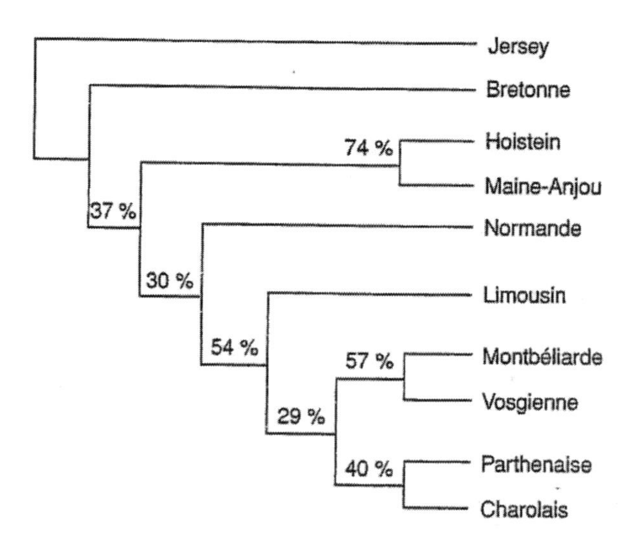

Figure 1. Phylogeny of 10 French breeds of cattle (from Moazami-Goudarzi et al., 1997). The tree is constructed from distances based on 17 molecular markers (microsatellites). The figures shown ("bootstrap" values) are percentages of occurrence of each node over 500 re-samplings.

This is a recursive definition, since $V(S_i)$ must also be calculated according to the same definition as V(S), i. e. $V(S_i)$ = maximum over S_i of $[d_{ij} + V(S_{ij})]$, d_{ij} being here defined as the distance between breed j and the subset S_{ij} obtained by excluding breeds i and j, and so on.

The appealing properties of this function and its applications in the context of farm livestock diversity have been described by Thaon d'Arnoldi *et al.* (1998). It can be mentioned that the solution of (3) also generates a phylogenetic tree which has the property of maximising the likelihood of the observed diversity, and whose reliability may be statistically assessed without re-sampling. In addition, the total branch length of the tree equals the V function defined in (3), and the length of each breed branch measures approximately the contribution of the corresponding breed to the total diversity V. An example of partitioning of diversity contributions among some European breeds of pigs is shown in Figure 2.

Contrary to the trees obtained by the usual algorithms (Hartl et Clark, 1997, p. 368), the branch lengths of the Weitzman tree do not require any evolutionary hypothesis. As stressed by Weitzman (quoted by Thaon d'Arnoldi *et al.*, 1998), diversity may be evaluated, and phylogenetic trees constructed, even though no evolutionary process underlies the relative positions of the elements of the set S.

Whatever the method used to construct trees, these allow *clustering* breeds into more or less distinct subsets. Clustering evidently depends on the hypotheses underlying the tree construction, and its reliability reflects the trees reliability. Other methods may be applied, as for instance correspondence analysis of breed × allele contingency tables. With such a method a set of breeds is represented in a Euclidean space, and the inertia of the system may then be taken as a measure of diversity (see Laloë *et al.*, 1999). This clustering process is free from any hypothesis about the evolutionary mechanism which has led to the diversity observed.

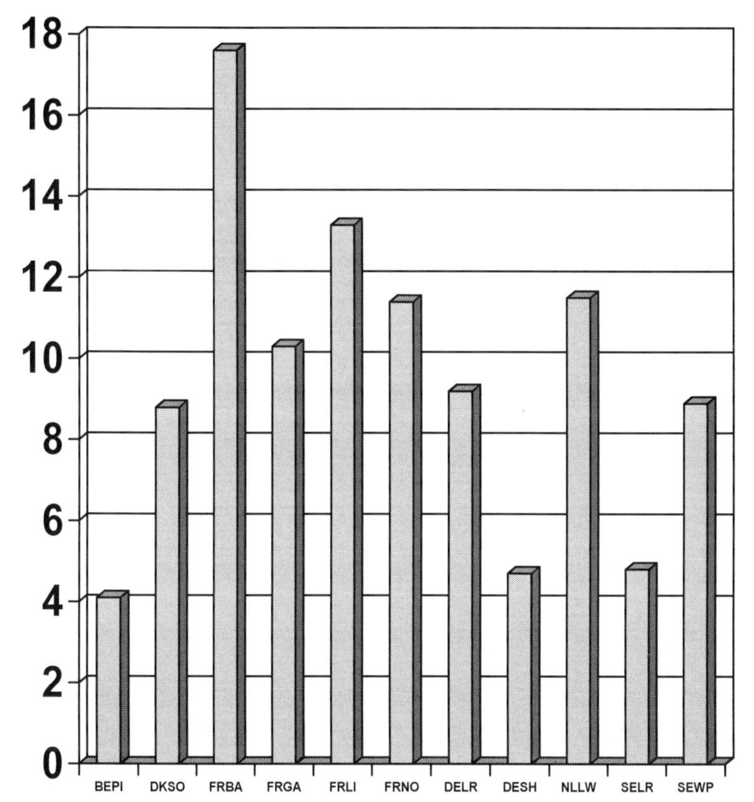

Figure 2. Marginal losses of diversity attached to eleven European breeds of pig (from Laval et al., 2000). Percentages show how much diversity reduction, relative to the eleven breeds diversity, is incurred when each breed is removed from the whole set. Breed code: Belgian Piétrain = BEPI, Danish Sortbroget (local breed) = DKSO, French Basque (local breed) = FRBA, French Gascon (local breed) = FRGA, French Limousin (local breed) = FRLI, French Normand (local breed) = FRNO, German Landrace = DELR, German Schwäbisch-Hällisches Schwein (local breed) = DESH, Dutch Large White = NLLW, Swedish Landrace = SELR, European wild pig = SEWP.

Within-breed genetic variability and allelic richness

We have so far considered characterising diversity by measures of sub-population differentiation, leaving aside measures of within-sub-population variability, which also deserve being taken into account. From that point of view, though heterozygosity is a classical criterion, several reasons may justify a complementary criterion such as the number of alleles present per locus in each sub-population (see Barker, 2001). In the study of Petit *et al.* (1998), the concept of *allelic richness* has been extended to the case of subdivided populations, in a parallel manner to heterozygosities. Petit *et al.* (1998) estimate the contribution of each sub-population to heterozygosity as the difference between the heterozygosity of the whole population and that obtained after excluding the sub-population considered. The contribution of each sub-population to the total allelic richness (C_T) is calculated similarly and may be partitioned into a contribution related to within-sub-population allelic richness (C_S) and a contribution related to its divergence from the other sub-populations (C_D). The example of the argan tree of Morocco (Petit *et al*., 1998), as re-analysed by Barker (2001), shows that the C_T and C_D contributions are strongly correlated with each other (0,86), while not being significantly correlated with the contribution to gene differentiation G_{ST} (Table 1). One also sees that, among the various contributions to allelic richness, only C_D is significantly related to the contribution to Weitzman diversity (D_W), while the latter is significantly correlated with G_{ST}.

Table 1. Correlations between various measures of diversity (from Barker, 2001). (12 subpopulations of argan tree of Morocco analysed by Petit et al., *1998; significant correlations are in bold).*

	G_{ST}	C_T	C_S	C_D
C_T	-0.05			
C_S	**-0.77**	0.47		
C_D	0.39	**0.86**	-0.05	
D_W	**0.66**	0.44	-0.21	**0.62**

G_{ST}, C_T, C_S, C_D and D_W are defined as the subpopulation contributions to diversity measured as follows:
G_{ST}: *gene differentiation* of Nei (defined in text).
C_T, C_S, C_D: total (T), within- (S) and between subpopulations (D) *allelic richness*.
D_W: *diversity function* of Weitzman.

This example suggests that between and within diversities are not necessarily related and that both should be taken into account. One also sees that allelic richness among sub-populations may help measuring their differentiation.

It is worth mentioning that this criterion of allelic richness, still seldom used in livestock breeds, is strongly dependent on sample size. It can indeed easily be predicted that, all things being equal otherwise, the number of alleles found in a breed will increase with the size of the sample examined. The method proposed by Petit *et al.* (1998) for eliminating this bias is to calculate a "corrected" allelic richness, which is the value expected in the smallest sample met over the set of sub-populations compared. One may however question whether such a "levelling down" procedure makes an optimal use of the information available.

Discussion and conclusions

The characterisation of genetic resources is a field of investigation which has recently seen a renewal of interest. The large number and the variety of methods and techniques which are available is often a source of puzzlement if not confusion. To the multiplicity of distance measures one must add the numerous methods of tree reconstruction, and the uncertainties surrounding their interpretation. It is now generally recognized that the phylogenetic processes behind domestic animal breeds have not much in common with those at work in wild species or sub-species, as noted for instance by Grosclaude *et al.* (1990) or Thaon d'Arnoldi *et al.* (1998). It is therefore risky to transpose to farm animals the methods which have initially been developed for natural populations. And one may wonder whether we have not too often failed to see the "forest" (of farm animal diversity) for the "trees" (of phylogeny).

For a long time, the way to optimise experimental designs for characterising a set of breeds has not received a proper attention. The recommendations of a working group convened by FAO in 1993 (Barker *et al.* 1998) were therefore particularly welcome. This group chose to base its recommendations on a distance measure (D) having a sampling variance V(D) particularly simple. Given the number n of individuals sampled per breed, the number L of loci, the number k of independent distances which may be calculated per locus, corresponding to k+1 alleles, and the true distance d, its sampling variance can be written:

$$V(D)=2[d+(1/n)]^2/Lk. \quad (4)$$

The formal demonstration of equation (4), presented by Foulley and Hill (1999), is based on the distance of Balakrishnan and Sanghvi (1968), itself akin to the distance of Reynolds *et al.* (1983). Formula (4) clearly integrates the variation resulting from both the sampling of individuals (n) in the population and the sampling of the marker loci (L) in the genome. The variances of the other measures of distance have generally more complex expressions (see, for instance, Laval, 1997).

Formula (4) enabled the FAO working group to recommend n=25 and Lk=50 for a sufficiently accurate evaluation of distances among breeds tightly related, i. e. d = 0.05. Formula (4) also shows that the number of loci L (or the number of independent alleles Lk) is more important to consider than the number of individuals per breed n when aiming at an accurate distance. The diversity function of Weitzman being a sum of distances, its accuracy may be calculated from equation (4). This could be a basis for a joint optimisation of the number of breeds and sample size per breed.

It is also worth mentioning that the statistical reliability of distances, though necessary to obtain significant phylogenies, does not guarantee they will automatically be obtained. The pig diversity study of Laval *et al.* (2000) may be used as an example. The distances estimated among the eleven breeds considered were all significant on the basis of formula (4), whereas no reliable phylogeny was obtained for nine of those breeds. And inversely, when doubtful phylogenies are obtained, as in Figure 1, one cannot conclude to an insufficient number of marker loci without a check on the sampling variance of the estimated distances and their statistical significance.

Acknowledgements

The authors are grateful to F. Grosclaude, (INRA, Génétique animale, Jouy-en-Josas) for the comments he provided during the preparation of this paper.

References

Balakrishnan, V. and L.D. Sanghvi, 1968. Distance between populations on the basis of attribute data. Biometrics 24, 859-865.

Barker, J.S.F., 2001. Conservation and management of genetic diversity: a domestic animal perspective. Can. J. For. Res. 31, 588-595.

Barker, J.S.F., W.G. Hill, D. Bradley, M. Nei, R. Fries and R.K. Wayne, 1998. Measurement of domestic animal diversity (MoDAD): original working group report. FAO, Rome.

BRG, 1999. Charte nationale pour la gestion des ressources génétiques. Bureau des Ressources Génétiques, Paris, 99 pp.

Cavalli-Sforza, L.L. and A.W.F. Edwards, 1967. Phylogenetic analysis: models and estimation procedures. Evolution 21, 550-570.

Chevalet, C., 1980. Calcul des coefficients d'identité, inégalités et distances génétiques. In :. Legay, J.M., Masson J.P and R. Tomassone (editors), Biométrie et Génétique, INRA, Paris, 42-49.
Felsenstein, J., 1985. Confidence limits on phylogenies : an approach using the bootstrap. Evolution 39, 783-791.
Foulley, J.-L. and W.G.Hill, 1999. On the precision of estimation of genetic distance. Genet. Sel. Evol. 31, 457-464.
Grosclaude, F., R.Y. Aupetit, J. Lefebvre and J.C. Mériaux, 1990. Essai d'analyse des relations génétiques entre les races bovines françaises à l'aide du polymorphisme biochimique. Genet. Sel. Evol. 22, 317-338.
Hartl, D.L. and A.G. Clark, 1997. Principles of Population Genetics (3rd Ed.). Sinauer Associates. Sunderland, Massachussetts, USA.
Laloë, D., K. Moazami-Goudarzi and P. Souvenir Zafindrajaona, 1999. Analyse des correspondances et biodiversité dans les races domestiques. Société Française de Biométrie, 20 mai 1999, Grenoble, 5pp.
Latter, B.D.H., 1972. Selection in finite populations with multiple alleles. III. Genetic divergence with centripetal selection and mutation. Genetics 70, 475-490.
Lauvergne, J.J., 1982. Genética en poblaciones animales despuès de la domesticacion : consecuencias para la conservacion de las razas. 2nd World Cong. Genet. Appl. Livestock Prod., 6, 77-87.
Laval, G., 1997. Modélisation et mesure de la différenciation génétique des races animales à l'aide de marqueurs microsatellites. DEA de Biologie des Populations, Génétique et Ecoéthologie, Université de Tours, 1997, 25pp.
Laval, G., N. Ianucelli, C. Legault, D. Milan, M.A.M. Groenen, L. Andersson, M. Fredholm, H. Geldermann, J.-L. Foulley, C. Chevalet and L. Ollivier, 2000. Genetic diversity of eleven European pig breeds. Genet. Sel. Evol. 32, 187-203.
Moazami-Goudarzi, K., D. Laloë, J.P. Furet and F.Grosclaude, 1997. Analysis of genetic relationships between 10 cattle breeds with 17 microsatellites. Anim. Genet. 28, 338-345.
Nei, M., 1973. Analysis of gene diversity in subdivided populations. Proc. Natl. Acad. Sci. USA 70, 3321-3323.
Nei, M., 1977. F-Statistics and analysis of gene diversity in subdivided populations. Ann. Hum. Genet. 41, 221-233.
Nei, M., 1987. Molecular Evolutionary Genetics. Columbia University Press, New York, USA.
Petit, R.J., A. El Mousadik and O. Pons, 1998. Identifying populations for conservation on the basis of genetic markers. Conserv. Biol. 12, 844-855.
Prevosti, A., J. Ocana and G. Alonso, 1975. Distances between populations of *Drosophila subobscura* based on chromosomal rearrangements. Theoret. Appl. Genet. 45, 231-241.
Reynolds, J., B.S. Weir and C.C. Cockerham, 1983. Estimation of the coancestry coefficient: basis for a short-term genetic distance. Genetics 105, 767-779.
Robert, C., 1992. L'analyse statistique bayésienne. Economica, Paris.
Rogers, J.S., 1972. Measures of genetic similarity and genetic distances. University of Texas Publ. 7213, 145-153.
Thaon d'Arnoldi,C., J.-L. Foulley and L. Ollivier, 1998. An overview of the Weitzman approach to diversity. Genet. Sel. Evol. 30, 149-161.
Weitzman, M.L., 1993. What to preserve ? An application of diversity theory to crane conservation. Quarter. J. Econ. 108, 157-183.

Appendix Some genetic distances used in genetics

-Notation :

- locus i = 1, 2,..I

- allele j = 1, 2,.., J_i (J_i is the number of alleles at locus i)

- allele frequencies x_{ij} and y_{ij} in the two populations considered.

-Rogers (1972) (Euclidian) : $D_R = \frac{1}{I}\sum_{i=1}^{I}\left[\frac{1}{2}\sum_{j=1}^{J_i}(x_{ij}-y_{ij})^2\right]^{1/2}$

-Prevosti *et al.* (1975) or Gregorius (Manhattan): $C_p = \frac{1}{2I}\left(\sum_{i=1}^{I}\sum_{j=1}^{J_i}|x_{ij}-y_{ij}|\right)$

-Cavalli-Sforza & Edwards (1967) (length of a chord) : $D_C = \frac{2}{\pi I}\sum_{i=1}^{I}\left[2(1-\sum_{j=1}^{J_i}x_{ij}y_{ij})\right]^{1/2}$

-Balakrishnan & Sanghvi (1968) (« Chi-square »): $X^2 = \frac{1}{J_+ - I}\sum_{i=1}^{I}\sum_{j=1}^{J_i}\frac{2(x_{ij}-y_{ij})^2}{x_{ij}+y_{ij}}$

-Reynolds *et al.* (1983) or F_{ST} of Latter (1972): $F_{ST} = \frac{1}{2}\frac{\sum_{i=1}^{I}\sum_{j=1}^{J_i}(x_{ij}-y_{ij})^2}{\sum_{i=1}^{I}\left(1-\sum_{j=1}^{J_i}x_{ij}y_{ij}\right)}$

-Nei M. (1987) (Molecular Evolutionary Genetics, Columbia University Press, New York) :

$$J_{XY} = I^{-1}\sum_{i=1}^{I}\sum_{j=1}^{J_i}x_{ij}y_{ij} ; J_X = I^{-1}\sum_{i=1}^{I}\sum_{j=1}^{J_i}x_{ij}^2$$

-Nei minimum: $D_m = \frac{1}{2I}\sum_{i=1}^{I}\sum_{j=1}^{J_i}(x_{ij}-y_{ij})^2 = (J_X + J_Y)/2 - J_{XY}$

-Nei standard: $D = -\ell n\frac{J_{XY}}{(J_X J_Y)^{1/2}}$

-Nei D_A: $D_A = 1 - \frac{1}{I}\sum_{i=1}^{I}\sum_{j=1}^{J_i}(x_{ij}y_{ij})^{1/2}$

NB : the F_{ST} distance can also be written using Nei's notation : $F_{ST} = \frac{(J_X + J_Y)/2 - J_{XY}}{1 - J_{XY}}$

A review on the methods of parentage and inbreeding analysis with molecular markers

B. Langlois

INRA-CRJ-SGQA, 78352 Jouy-en-Josas – France

Abstract

In horse populations there is a great concern for pedigree. Genetic markers are commonly used for exclusion procedures to assess the right sire and dam of the foal. However pedigree information is limited because the total genetic history of an animal or a population can not be traced from the beginning. In this paper we try to review how genetic markers can help us to overcome these difficulties. Formulae in the literature for estimating F from the state of markers consider the two causes that make sorting two genes alike. They are either identical by descent or alike in state. All authors agree that estimators for pairwise relatedness or individual inbreeding coefficients need a lot of independent co-dominant marker loci where alleles are balanced in frequencies in order to reach a minimum accuracy in estimations. In this perspective the development of a kit of SNP satisfying these conditions would be a tool of great interest to address the problems connected with parentage inbreeding and genetic diversity in horse populations where the good management of pedigree information appears insufficient to do it properly.

Keywords: genetic markers, parentage, inbreeding, horse

Introduction

In horse populations there is a great concern for pedigree. Most of stud-books started during the 19th century and some of them even earlier. This administrative work was done very carefully as it was done for humans with parish register. However this did not exclude some errors which justified the use of genetic markers in routine procedure as early as the 1970s. Now genetic markers are systematically used for breeds such as arab, thoroughbred and trotter and commonly used for the others in the case of artificial insemination or at random to discourage fraud. The result is a very low percentage of parentage errors in horse breeding. Genetic markers in horse breeding are only used for exclusion procedures to assess the right sire and dam of the foal. Categorical allocation to select the most likely parent from a foal of non-excluded parents is not practised for legal reasons. However pedigree information is limited because the total genetic history of an animal or a population can not be traced from the beginning. Even with very complete and reliable pedigrees, there are still events in the past which are not described like bottlenecks or real number of unrelated founders. In this paper we try to review how genetic markers can help us to overcome these difficulties.

Exclusion

The earliest conceptually simplest technique of parentage analysis is exclusion. This technique based on Mendelian rules of inheritance uses incompatibilities between parents and offspring to reject particular parent-offspring hypotheses. It was used a low scale for a long time in horse breeding: two chestnut (ee) parents are expected to have only chestnut foals (ee). One grey foal (G-) is expected to have at least one grey parent (G-)' which can be generalised for each recessive allele (black E-/aa) or dominant one (bai E-/A-).

More generally a foal can not receive an allele which is not present in his parents. One sees immediately that co-dominant loci where genotype of foal and parents will appear will be more efficient that dominant/recessive ones for that technique.

Exclusion is an appealing approach because exclusions of all but one parent pair from a complete sample of all possible parents for each offspring in a population could be considered the paragon of parentage analysis. However it is limited by the occurrence of typing errors and at a lower rate of mutations. The list of markers used for exclusion also plays a major role. Jamieson and Taylor (1997), Dodds *et al.*(1996) made a thorough analysis of these questions. It is concluded that the exclusion probability increases with the number of loci that can be used as genetic markers, with the number of alleles at each locus and with the evenness of the allele frequency at each locus (Chakraborty *et al.*1974, Selvin (1980),Ryman and Chakraborty (1982), Smouse and Chakraborty (1986). However the relationship exhibits a diminishing marginal return because an additional marker applies its power of exclusion only on non-excluded parents before its application.

This can be generalised to other types of exclusion. For an autosomal marker first, it is always easier to detect incorrect offspring assignments (i.e. when mating pairs are known) than other types of exclusion and second, paternity (or maternity) exclusion is greater with the other parent known than unknown as expected.

For daughters the X- linked markers always has a greater exclusions probability no matter what situation is being tested except for maternity testing without knowledge of the sire where the autosomal and X- linked markers have the same exclusion probability). For sons the autosomal marker has higher exclusion probability except for maternity testing in which case, the X linked marker would be better.

The importance of exclusion probability to paternity assignment is that an increase in the exclusion probability increases the probability of paternity among the set of non-excluded parents. Clearly the likelihood of choosing the correct non-excluded parent increase. In the extreme case, as the exclusion probability approaches 1, most progeny can be assigned exclusively to a single male or female parent in the population.

It may also be desirable to require exclusion at more than one locus to reduce the effect of possible genotyping errors, mutation or of unknown null alleles.

Table 1 shows the exclusion probability of eleven microsatellites markers routinely used for parentage control in horse breeding in France. The exclusion probability for thoroughbred and Arab breeds is now reaching near one value (Amigues *et al.* 2000). With older systems (9, haemolytic, 24 aglutination and 10 electrophoretic) it was only of 0.952 for thoroughbred and 0.954 for arab. These now very high exclusion probabilities were recently confirmed by Cho and Cho (2004) for Korean native horses.

As it can be inferred from the studies in horses 10 to 20 polymorphic loci allow probabilities of exclusion close to 1. The paragon of parentage analysis is therefore reached for horse populations. For each foal the right sire and dam can be assigned.

Table 1. Exclusion probabilities in two breeds for routine microsatellites markers used in France (source: Amigues et al. 2000).

Microsatellites			Thoroughbred		Arab	
Name	Origin	Reference	Alleles number	Exclusion Probability	Alleles number	Exclusion probability
AHT4	U.K.	Binns *et al.* 1995	6	0.49	7	0.57
AHT5	U.K.	Binns *et al.* 1995	6	0.51	6	0.45
ASB2	Australia	Breen *et al.* 1997	8	0.68	8	0.37
HMS1	France	Guérin *et al.* 1994	4	0.35	6	0.36
HMS3	France	Guérin *et al.* 1994	6	0.35	6	0.46
HMS6	France	Guérin *et al.* 1994	7	0.32	6	0.46
HMS7	France	Guérin *et al.* 1994	5	0.58	7	0.53
HTG4	Sweden	Ellegren *et al.* 1992	5	0.25	6	0.41
HTG6	Sweden	Ellegren *et al.* 1992	7	0.33	7	0.37
HTG10	Sweden	Marklund *et al.* 1994	7	0.54	8	0.53
VHL20	The Netherlands	Van Haeringen *et al.* 1994	7	0.50	10	0.62
	Total probability of identity		68	0.9989	77	0.9991
			$4.6\ 10^{-10}$		$1.8\ 10^{-10}$	

Allocation or assignment

If complete exclusion is not possible it is often not sufficient to derive accurate population statistics on mating patterns. Consequently techniques were developed that assigned progeny to non-excluded parents based on likelihood scores derived from their genotypes. According to Jones and Ardren (2003) these techniques assign offspring either categorically or fractionally.

Categorical allocation uses likelihood-based approaches (Meagher and Thompson, 1987) to select the most likely parent from a pool of non-excluded parents. This method involves calculating the logarithm of the likelihood ratio (LOD score) by dividing the likelihood of an individual (or pair of individuals being the parent (or parents) of a given offspring by the likelihood of these individuals being unrelated. After an exhaustive evaluation of all possible parents, the offspring are assigned to the parent (or parental pair) with the highest LOD score. When all-parent offspring relationships show zero likelihood, offspring are unassigned. Parentage remains also ambiguous when multiple parent-offspring relationships obtain high no zero likelihood. Contrary to strict exclusion methods, likelihood-based allocation method, because it is based on the evaluation of a probability, allows for some degree of transmission errors due to misreading or mutation (SanCristobal and Chevalet 1997).

It is also for this reason that allocation techniques are not acepted in horse breeding. For forensic purpose you need to establish true facts and not only their probabilities. However limiting yourself to true facts limits the amount of information used. Allocations techniques remain therefore appealing because they allow a better use of the available information in statistical terms.

Returning to Meagher's and Thompson's (1987) original proposition for categorical allocation. In all cases we examine genotypes, g_A, g_B and g_O at a single autosomal locus for three individuals (O, B and A). Assuming unlinked loci, information from multiple loci can be combined by summing the LOD scores over all loci. Transition probabilities (T) for use of the following equations can be found in Marshall *et al.* (1998)for co-dominant markers and in Gerber *et al.* (2000) for dominant markers. Three main cases have to be examined:

a) Identifying one parent when the other is known. Letting B represent the known parent and A the alleged parent, the LOD score for A being the parent of O is:

$$\text{LOD score (A parent of O)} = \text{Log}_e \frac{T(g_O \mid g_B, g_A)}{T(g_O \mid g_B)}$$

Where $T(g_O|g_B,g_A)$ is the transition probability of g_O given g_B and g_A and $T(g_O|g_B)$ is the transition probability of g_O given g_B.

b) Identifying one parent with no information about the other parent. In this case, no information is available concerning parentage of O. The single parent LOD score for B being the parent of O is:

$$\text{LOD score (B parent of O)} = \text{Log}_e \frac{T(g_O \mid g_B)}{P(g_O)}$$

Where $P(g_O)$ is the frequency of the offspring's genotype in the population.

c) Identifying a parental pair starting with no prior information. Parental pair allocation is an approach for identifying parent-offspring relationships by constructing genotypic triplets consisting of a proposed offspring and proposed maternal and paternal parents. This procedure involves calculating a breeding likelihood, which is defined as the likelihood of a parental pair producing the multi locus genotype found in the offspring being examined. The breeding likelihood of a given offspring on the basis of a single locus is:

$$\text{LOD score (A, B parent of O)} = \text{Log}_e \frac{T(g_O \mid g_A, g_B)}{P(g_O)}$$

The fractional allocation method assigns some function, between 0 and 1, for each offspring to all non-excluded candidate parents. The proportion of an offspring allocated to a particular candidate parent is proportional to its likelihood of parenting the offspring compared to all other non-excluded candidate parents. Single parent and parent pair likelihoods are calculated in the same way as in the categorical allocation method (Devlin *et al.*, 1988). Because the fractional technique splits an offspring among all compatible males it is guaranteed to be incorrect from a biological standpoint, an offspring having only one father and one mother. However for the study of particular problems connected with reproductive success in natural populations this method proved his statistical superiority. Indeed, the categorical allocation by the most likely method as formulated above embodies some bias in that the most likely parent will always be that individual in the population that has the highest number of loci homozygous for the necessary paternal gamete contribution that complements the maternal ones. It was also emphasised by Thompson and Meagher (1987) that bilateral relatives such as full sibs may be more likely parents than the true parent individuals.

We will also see further that maximum likelihood techniques are asymptotically optimal but can prove to be very inaccurate for a low number of markers.

First conclusion on exclusion and allocation

For horse breeding we are now in a situation where the exclusion probability of the microsatellites markers routinely in use is close to one for all breeds. Therefore the allocation techniques decrease in interest at least to identify the first generation parents (Sire and Dam) to certify the pedigree. To ascertain sire and dam of an offspring when done, over several generations, makes the information of pedigree very reliable.

However this is not sufficient to ascertain exact genetic relationships between individuals of a population when some errors in the past (Kavar *et al.*, 2002) and when the assumption of unrelated founders (ancestors without known parents) can not be accepted as it is mainly the case in horse populations (Mahon and Cunningham, 1982, MacCluer *et al.*, 1983, Cothran *et al.*, 1984, Moureaux *et al.*, 1996, Cunningham *et al.*, 2001, Zechner *et al.*, 2002).

We can also remark that a sire or a dam transmit half of his alleles to his offspring with certainty, this is only the case in probability for other relationships as shown Table 2. One can want to check the realisation of this probability with genetic markers particularly when panmixia is not realised in the case of inbreeding selection and homogamy.

Table 2. Cotterham's K values for some standard genealogical relationships, in the absence of inbreeding Source: Thompson (1975).

Relationship of A to B	K_0	K_1	K_2
Unrelated	1	0	0
Offspring, parent	0	1	0
Sib	1/4	1/2	1/4
Identical twin	0	0	1
Niece, nephew, uncle, aunt			
Grandparent, grand-child	1/2	1/2	0
Half-sib			
First-cousin, parent's half-sib, half-sib's child	3/4	1/4	0
Double first cousin	9/16	6/16	1/16
Half-sibs whose non-identical parents are:			
1- sibs or parent-offspring	3/8	1/2	1/8
2- half-sibs	7/16	1/2	1/16

K_0, K_1, K_2 being the probability of 0, 1 and 2 genes in common
Other relationships have $K_1 \leq 1/2$ and $K_2 \leq 1/16$

Short history of the description of genetic pairwise relationships

Cotterman 1940 first introduced the k coefficients probability that two non-inbred individuals have 0, 1 or 2 genes in common. These are sufficient specification of the relationship between any two non-inbred individual. Malécot 1948 extended this work introducing the parentage coefficient between two individuals. This is the probability of drawing two genes identical by descent in each individual. Consequently the inbreeding coefficient of an individual, the probability that the two genes of a same locus are identical by descent is the parentage coefficient of his parents. This allowed a more thorough use of pedigree information. Wright (1943) defined the kinship coefficient r, as the correlation between uniting gametes. That is two times Malécot's parentage coefficient The last step of description of pairwise relationships was given by Jacquard (1972) for two individuals at one locus nine situations of identity were distinguished according to Figure 1.

Figure 1. Scheme of the nine situations of identity according to Jacquard 1972.

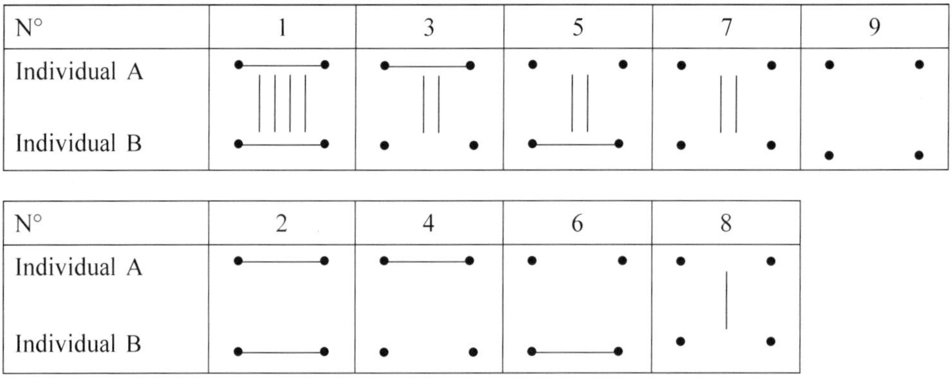

N°	1	3	5	7	9
Individual A					
Individual B					

N°	2	4	6	8
Individual A				
Individual B				

According to these nine situations a probability Δ_i is given according to the pedigree and we have the following relations with inbreeding coefficient f and the parentage coefficient φ.

$$f_A = \Delta_1 + \Delta_2 + \Delta_3 + \Delta_4$$
$$f_B = \Delta_1 + \Delta_2 + \Delta_5 + \Delta_6$$
$$\varphi_{AB} = \Delta_1 + \frac{1}{2}(\Delta_3 + \Delta_5 + \Delta_7) + \frac{1}{4}\Delta_8$$

The correspondence with Cotterman's coefficients is:
K_0 in situations 2 4 6 and 9 (0 gene in common for A and B)
K_1 in situations 8 3 5 (1 gene in common)
K_2 in situations 1 and 7 (2 genes in common)

How to infer the estimation of f or φ .from the situation of genetic markers identity

We must go back to Malécot (1948) to define the two concepts that makes two alleles at the same locus alike. They are either "identical by descent" (IBD) or "alike in state" (AIS). He wrote therefore the probability s_{ii} of being homozygote for allele i equals the probability of being IBD defined as the inbreeding coefficient multiplied by the probability of drawing the i allele, plus the probability (1-f) of not being IBD multiplied by the probability of drawing at random twice the same allele (probability of being AIS):

$$s_{ii} = fp_i + (1-f)p_i^2 = fp_i + (1-p_i) + p_i^2$$

The probability s_{ij} of being heterozygote for alleles i and j equals the probability of not being IBD multiplied by the probability of drawing at random i and j or j and i.

$$s_{ij} = (1\text{-}f)2p_ip_j$$

Where p_i is the frequency of allele i. The probability of being homozygous at the locus is derived:

$$\sum_i s_{ii} = f + (1-f)\sum_i p_i^2 \qquad (1)$$

or

$$\sum_i s_{ii} = f(1-\sum_i p_i^2) + \sum_i p_i^2$$

And the probability of being heterozygous:

$$\sum_{i \neq j} s_{ij} = 1 - \sum_i s_{ii}$$

$$= 1 - \sum_i p_i^2 - f(1-\sum_i p_i^2)$$

$$\left(1-\sum_i s_{ii}\right) = (1-f)\left(1-\sum_i p_i^2\right)$$

From the knowledge of p_i and the observed s_{ii} or s_{ij} f can be estimated. This formula is presented many times in the literature under different forms considering f or parentage coefficients φ of the parents, multi- or bi-allelism. Let us cite Wright (1978)analogous formulae for subdivided population discussed by Malécot (1969):

$$(1-F_{IT}) = (1-F_{IS})(1-F_{ST})$$

where according to Eding (2002) or Robertson and Hill (1984) F_{IT} is defined as the total kinship between two individuals within the whole subdivided population. F_{IS} is the kinship between two individuals within a subpopulation and can be extracted from the (limited) pedigree information, $F_{IS} = f$. F_{ST} is the correlation between random gametes from the same sub population relative to the whole population: $F_{ST} = 1 - H_S/H_T$.
H_s is the heterozygosity intra subpopulation
H_t is the heterozygosity for the whole population

Let us also cite Lynch (1988) formula:

$$f = \frac{\sum_i s_{ii} - \sum_i p_i^2}{1-\sum_i p_i^2}$$

(see equation (1) probability of being homozygous)

All techniques of estimating pairwise relationships from the state of molecular markers derive from this approach. They can be applied at the individual level or at the intra- and between-population levels. However, one can immediately anticipate how low will be the accuracy of the one locus approach. We are therefore inclined to propose a multi-locus approach.

Multi-locus approach

For the choice of an adequate and efficient set of markers the weighting of information of each locus plays a major role for determining best statistical estimators (Ritland, 1996) and also for the choice of efficient and adequate markers. Indeed, one can easily understand that fixed loci will not give any information on parentage and that at the opposite loci with more balanced frequencies will do it.

From a statistical standpoint (Ritland, 1996) one problem in estimating relatedness or inbreeding for individual is statistical bias caused by small samples. In considering sample size, there are two dimensions the number of individuals, and the number of marker loci. The number of individuals if considered alone is at a bare minimum of one for inbreeding, two for relatedness, magnifying the bias due to small samples, even when a large number of marker loci are used. This can be a significant problem when using maximum likelihood estimators which are often recognized to show bias with small sample sizes. However individuals or mating pairs are not isolated they belong to a population or a sub-population. Indeed, the parentage coefficient of two individuals and therefore the inbreeding of an individual have no meaning per se. The concept takes sense only when it is related to a population or a subpopulation constituting the gene pool. This question about the number of individuals can therefore be partly translated on the problem of estimating allele frequencies in these populations. It will give the basis for the genotypic probabilities of randomly chosen animals. Deviations from this basis will serve for parentage analysis. Without reference there is no measurement possible.

Method of Moment Estimator (MME)

Generality

Its primary advantage is the reduction of bias with individual level estimates and a lack of distributional assumptions.

To describe the data we denote S_i as the observed proportion of pairs similar for marker allele i. It can be regarded as an indicator variable of relationship. For the case of inbreeding coefficient f, then $S_i = 1$ if the two alleles at a locus are allele i ; otherwise $S_i = 0$. For the case of two-individual relatedness φ, there are four equally probable ways of sampling two alleles, two for each two relatives. Si is the average over the four ways that a given pair of alleles can be sampled.

For individual A: $S_i = 1$ for the situation 1, 2, 3 and 4.of Jacquard (1972) $S_i = 0$ for the others.

For individual B: $S_i = 1$ for the situations 1, 2, 5 and 6. $S_i = 0$ for the others.

For the pair of individual A and B we have defined $S_i = \frac{1}{4}(I_{11} + I_{12} + I_{21} + I_{22})$. Therefore:

$S_i = 1$ for the situation 1,
$S_i = ½$ for the situations 3, 5 and 7,
$S_i = ¼$ for the situation 8,
$S_i = 0$ for the situations 2, 4, 6 and 9.

The expectation of S_i (denoted s_i) conditioned upon relationship, is as we have seen:

$$s_i = \rho p_i + (1-\rho)p_i^2, \qquad \text{(1bis)}$$

Where ρ is the two-gene relationship, which equals either f or φ. This expectation assumes the population gene frequencies equal the pedigree gene frequencies (the gene pool from which alleles were randomly drawn during the formation of the pedigree. The probabilities over several independent loci are the product of these single-locus probabilities.

Correlation method (Ritland, 1996)

To obtain an efficient method of moments estimator (MME) for two-gene relationship, one first obtains estimates for each marker allele i, for i=1 to n (the number of alleles at the locus), based upon the observation of whether the alleles are both of type i or not. Although there are n(n+1)/2 combinations of alleles each of which can give an estimate of relationship, these estimates are not independent, and only the set of n estimates corresponding to the sharing of allele i, i=1, n, are sufficient to capture all information in the data (Robertson and Hill, 1984). The variance-covariance matrix of these n estimates is then used to optimally combine the n estimates in a linear fashion into a single estimate.

By equating observed quantities to their expectations in (1bis), we obtain an estimator for each allele i at an n-allele locus as:

$$\hat{\rho}_i = \frac{S_i - P_i^2}{P_i Q_i}, i = 1, ..., n \tag{2}$$

where P_i = 1 - Q is the estimate of gene frequency p_i (capital letters are used to denote estimated quantities), and the hat denotes the estimate. For simplicity, gene frequency can be estimated by collecting alleles in the entire sampled population (this assumes low mean relationship).

The total estimate of relationship (relatedness or inbreeding is then the weighted average:

$$\hat{\rho} = \sum_i w_i \hat{\rho}_i \tag{3}$$

Where the weights w_i sum to unity.

To obtain the optimal weights, note that the n estimates of relationship (2) have variances and covariances:

$$\text{var}(\hat{\rho}_i) = \frac{s_i(1-s_i)}{cp_i^2 q_i^2}$$

$$\text{Cov}(\hat{\rho}_i \hat{\rho}_j) = \frac{-s_i s_j}{cp_i p_j q_i q_j}, \text{ i, j} = 1, 2, ..., n$$

These are obtained by noting that the S_i are multinomially distributed with variances $s_i(1-s_i)$ and covariances - $s_i s_j$, and that Var(aX+b) = a^2Var(x) for a and b constant. The constant c=1 for f while C≤4 for φ; its exact value is irrelevant because it cancels when computing weights.

The optimal weights are then found via a standard procedure of weighting correlated estimates.

Briefly these weights minimize $Var(\hat{\rho}) = w^T V w$ where w is an n element column vector of weights and V is the variance – covariance matrix of allele- specific estimates.

Unless one assumes a prior of $\rho=0$ or $\rho=1$ the expression of w must be solved numerically.

Then multi-locus estimates of relatedness involve a second stage of weighting. After a weighted estimate is found for each locus, a "grand" weighted estimate is found by weighting estimates across loci. If loci are unlinked and in linkage equilibrium, estimates from different loci will be independent and the weighting used for a given locus is simply proportional to the inverse of its variance as computed by the above weighting procedure.

A simple simplified MME estimator can be obtained by assuming $\rho=0$ in the weights. The procedure for obtaining optimal weights gives for allele i $w_i = q_i/(n-1)$ for n number of alleles at the locus. This gives an estimator for a single locus, which combines information along alleles, as

$$\hat{\rho} = \sum_i \frac{S_i - P_i^2}{(n-1)P_i}$$

To combine estimates among loci, we use the fact that at zero true relationship and known gene frequency, the variance of single locus weighted MME is proportional to 1/(n-1), regardless of the frequency distribution of alleles. The inverse of this quantity serves as the weight. This gives a simplified multi locus estimator of relationship, based upon a prior ρ of zero as:

$$\hat{\rho} = \sum_{i,\ell} \frac{S_{i\ell} - P_{i\ell}^2}{P_{i\ell}} / \sum_{\ell}(n_\ell - 1)$$

where ℓ denotes the locus. This estimator was first described by Li and Horvitz (1953).

A second simple method of moment estimator for ρ can be obtained by assuming $\rho=1$ in the weights. The weights then become $p_i q_i/(1-J)$, for J the expected homozygosity. Over m independent loci, this estimator equals:

$$\hat{\rho} = \frac{S-J}{1-J}$$

for $J = \frac{1}{m}\sum_{i,\ell} P_{i\ell}^2$ the mean expected homozygosity over the m loci and $S = \frac{1}{m}\sum_{i,\ell} S_{i\ell}$ the arithmetic average of allele similarity between the two individuals across loci.

Simulation results showed the variance of the MME to be approximately a function of 1/m for m the number of loci. However for relationships spanning a wide range and for many different distributions of gene frequency a systematic bias on the order of 1/N was observed, for N the number of individuals used to estimate gene frequency. Greater efficiency is obtained by using loci with even gene frequencies. The estimation of MME almost plateaus by 40-60 individuals where it nearly equals the predicted asymptotic variance (1/[4(n-1)m] for n alleles at each of m loci.

Regression method

Lynch and Ritland (1999) pursuing their search for optimal estimators for common situations when the number of loci are under 50, changed the name MME in that of correlation method and proposed a new one on the same principles but based on a regression approach. They also refined their analyses in proposing estimators for "higher-order" coefficients. The relatedness (kinship) coefficient r for two individuals (A and B), two times their coefficient of coancestry (or parentage) φ can be written:

$$r = \frac{1}{2}k_1 + k_2$$

Where k_1 and k_2 are the Cotterham's coefficients of table2.

Consider a single locus with n alleles and let A be the reference individual (with alleles a and b) and B be the proband individual (with alleles c and d). The conditional probabilities for the n(n+1)/2 possible genotypes in B can be expressed as a function of k_1 and k_2 and the known allele frequencies:

$$\begin{aligned} P(y = cd \mid x = ab) = {} & P_0(cd).(1 - k_1 - k_2) \\ & + P_1(cd \mid ab).k_1 + P_2(cd \mid ab).k_2 \end{aligned}$$

Where $P_0(cd)$ is the Hardy-Weinberg probability of genotype cd, and $P_1(cd|ab)$ and $P_2(cd|ab)$ denote the probabilities of genotype cd in B given genotype ab in A, the first being conditional on the two individuals having one gene identical by descent and the second being conditional on two genes being identical by descent.

Considering first A being homozygous for allele i and letting pi be the frequency of the ith allele, the preceding equation can be written:

$$\begin{aligned} P(ii \mid ii) &= p_i^2 + p_i(1 - p_i)k_1 + (1 - p_i^2)k_2 \\ P(i. \mid ii) &= 2p_i\,(1 - p_i) + (1 - p_i)(1 - 2p_i)k_1 \\ & \quad - 2p_i(1 - p_i)k_2 \end{aligned}$$

which can be rearranged to yield the following estimators:

$$\hat{k}_1 = \frac{(1 + p_i)\hat{P}(i. \mid ii) + 2p_i\hat{P}(ii \mid ii) - 2p_i}{(1 - p_i)^2}$$

$$\hat{k}_2 = \frac{p_i^2 - p_i\hat{P}(i. \mid ii) + (1 - 2p_i)\,\hat{P}(ii \mid ii)}{(1 - p_i)^2}$$

and,

$$\hat{r} = \frac{\hat{P}(i.|ii) + 2\hat{P}(ii|ii) - 2p_i}{2(1-p_i)}$$

P(i./ii) and P(ii/ii) are estimated as 0/1 variables. Both probabilities are 0 if the proband B has no alleles in common with the reference A. Thus for example when individual B contains 2, 1 and 0 i alleles the estimates of r are 1, (1-2pi)/2(1-pi) and –pi/(1-pi) respectively.

When A is heterozygous and the locus multiallelic there are six classes of conditional probabilities. Then the number of observed 0/1 variables exceeds the number of unknows (k_1 and k_2). To deal with this situation a weighted least-square approximation is provided.

A general one locus estimator which cover all the cases is best described by introducing "indicator variables" for the sharing of pairs of alleles:
As before let the reference individual A have the alleles a and b and the proband individual B alleles c and d. If the reference individual is homozygous, S_{ab}=1 while if it is heterozygous S_{ab}=0. Likewise if allele a from the reference individual is the same as allele c from the proband S_{ac}=1, while S_{ac}=0 if it is different. In total, there are six S's corresponding to the six ways of choosing two objects without replacement from a pool of four objects. Letting p_a, p_b be the frequencies of alleles a and b in the population, the fully general expressions for the two locus-specific coefficients of primary interest are:

$$\hat{r} = \frac{p_a(S_{bc} + S_{bd}) + p_b(S_{ac} + S_{ad}) - 4p_a p_b}{(1 + S_{ab})(p_a + p_b) - 4p_a p_b}$$

$$\hat{k}_2 = \frac{2p_a p_b - p_a(S_{bc} + S_{bd}) - p_b(S_{ac} + S_{ad}) + (S_{ac}S_{bd}) + (S_{ad}S_{bc})}{(1 + S_{ab})(1 - p_a - p_b) + 2p_a p_b}$$

There is no particular reason to use one member of a pair of individuals as the reference and the other as proband. Thus the reciprocal estimates rAB and rBA can be arithmetically averaged to further refine the pairwise relationship estimates.

Multilocus estimates

As shown before, with statistically independent marker loci the locus-specific weights that minimize the sampling variance of the overall estimates are simply the inverse of the sampling variance of the locus-specific estimates. Approximations can be obtained by assuming A and B unrelated and general expressions for the weights w(*l*) are given by:

$$w_{r,A}(\ell) = \frac{1}{\mathrm{Var}[\hat{r}(\ell)]} = \frac{(1 + S_{ab})(p_a + p_b) - 4p_a p_b}{2p_a p_b}$$

$$w_{k_2,A}(\ell) = \frac{1}{\mathrm{Var}\left[\hat{k}_2(\ell)\right]} = \frac{(1 + S_{ab})(1 - p_a - p_b) + 2p_a p_b}{2p_a p_b}$$

Other methods

Queller and Goodnight (1989) presented also a regression based estimator for two-gene relatedness. Their one locus estimator was designed to estimate relatedness within groups of individuals but it can be adapted for estimating pair wise relationships. However their estimator

$$\hat{r} = \frac{0.5(S_{ac} + S_{ad} + S_{bc} + S_{bd}) - p_a - p_b}{1 + S_{ab} - p_a - p_b}$$

has limited utility with diallelic loci. Indeed, if A is heterozygous then Sab=0 and the equation is undefined because $p_a + p_b = 1$

Eding and Meuwissen (2001) with similar approach and starting from Lynch's (1988) formula estimating f from the observed similarity S_ℓ at a locus ℓ and $h_\ell = \sum_{i=1}^{n\ell} p_{i,\ell}^2$ the probability of alleles of locus ℓ being AIS (alike in state), are writing:

$$\begin{aligned} E(S_\ell) &= P\ell \\ &= f + (1-f)h_\ell \\ &= h_\ell + (1-h_\ell)f \end{aligned} \qquad \text{(1 ter)}$$

This leads to the variance of $\hat{f}$

$$\text{var}(\hat{f}) = \frac{1}{(1-h_\ell)^2}\text{var}(S_\ell) \qquad (4)$$

Since S is the probability that two random alleles drawn from two individuals are alike, the distribution of S is binomial. The variance of S_ℓ for a locus ℓ is given as:

$$\text{var}(S_\ell) = P_\ell(1 - P_\ell) \qquad (5)$$

Filling (1 ter) in (5) yields

$$\begin{aligned} \text{Var}(S_\ell) &= f(1-h_\ell) + h_\ell - \left[f^2(1-h_\ell)^2 + 2fh_\ell + h_\ell^2\right] \\ &= f(1-h_\ell)(1-2h_\ell) + h_\ell(1-h_\ell) - f^2(1-h_\ell)^2 \end{aligned} \qquad (6)$$

Substitution of 6 in 4 gives:

$$\begin{aligned} \text{Var}(\hat{f}) &= \frac{f(1-h_\ell)(1-2h_\ell) + h_\ell(1-h_\ell) - f^2(1-h_\ell)^2}{(1-h_\ell)^2} \\ &= \frac{h_\ell + f(1-2h_\ell) - f^2(1-h_\ell)}{(1-h_\ell)} \end{aligned} \qquad (7)$$

An over all loci estimation of f can be obtained through averaging over m analysed loci. We may use the inverse of the variance of the estimates of f for each independent locus as weights. We obtain the following estimation:

$$f = \frac{\sum_{l=1}^{m} \hat{f}_\ell \left[\frac{(1-h_\ell)}{h_\ell + f(1-2h_\ell) - f^2(1-h_\ell)} \right]}{\sum_{l=1}^{m} \left[\frac{(1-h_\ell)}{h_\ell + f(1-2h_\ell) - f^2(1-h_\ell)} \right]} \quad (8)$$

Maximum Likelihood Estimator (MLE)

The maximum likelihood procedure was extensively investigated by Thompson (1975, 1976) for inferring pairwise relationship. She discussed the power of likelihood to distinguish among major types of relationships (parent-offspring, full sibs, half sibs, etc…) and unrelated. She found that due to large errors of inference it is difficult, even with 20 highly polymorphic loci, to distinguish among the major classes of relatives. However MLE gives asymptotically efficient estimates when the number of loci exceeds 50. This allows test of hypothesis via likelihood ratios and a better analytical analysis of the problem as we will try to demonstrate now.

The likelihood Y of the genotype of individual A for m independent loci is the product of the likelihood for each locus:

$$Y = \prod_{\ell=1}^{k} [h_\ell + (1-h_\ell) f_A] \times \prod_{\ell=1}^{j} (1-h_\ell)(1-f_A)$$

k loci being homozygous and j loci being heterozygous for individual A with f_A coefficient of inbreeding. h_ℓ being the probability of being homozygous for the locus ℓ in panmixia (equals the two alleles being AIS), $(1-h_\ell)$ being the probability of being heterozygous:

$$Y = (1+f_A)^k \prod_{\ell=1}^{k} \left[h_\ell \frac{(1-f_A)}{(1+f_A)} + \frac{f_A}{(1+f_A)} \right] \times (1-f_A)^j \prod_{\ell=1}^{j} (1-h_\ell)$$

Taking the natural logarithm:

$$\mathrm{Log_e}\, Y = k\, \mathrm{Log_e}\,(1+f_A) + \sum_{\ell=1}^{k} \mathrm{Log_e} \left[h_\ell \frac{(1-f_A)}{(1+f_A)} + \frac{f_A}{(1+f_A)} \right] + j\, \mathrm{Log_e}\,(1-f_A) + \sum_{\ell=1}^{j} \mathrm{Log_e}\,(1-h_\ell)$$

Derivative of $\mathrm{Log_e} Y$ with respect to f_A:

$$\frac{\partial\, \mathrm{Log_e}\, Y}{\partial f_A} = k \frac{1}{(1+f_A)} + \sum_{\ell=1}^{k} \frac{1-2h_\ell}{(1+f_A)[h_\ell + (1-h_\ell) f_A]} - j \frac{1}{1-f_A}$$

Which is zero for:

$$(1-f_A)\left\{\sum_{\ell=1}^{k}(1-\frac{2h_\ell-1}{[h_\ell+(1-h_\ell)f_A]})\right\}=j(1+f_A)$$

Defining $S_\ell=1$ for homozygotes and $S_\ell=0$ for heterozygotes we have for the $m=k+j$ loci

$$(1-f_A)\left\{\sum_{\ell=1}^{m}S_\ell(1-\frac{2h_\ell-1}{h_\ell+(1-h_\ell)f_A})\right\}=(1+f_A)\sum_{\ell=1}^{m}(1-S_\ell)$$

Considering S*l* taking the values 0 ¼ ½ 1, according to the situation of identity (see p7: generality) this formula allows the estimation of φ the parentage coefficient instead of f_A.
By definition of C and D

$$(1-f_A)\,C=(1+f_A)\,D$$

$$f_A=\frac{C-D}{C+D}$$

One can note that for

$$h_\ell=\sum_{i=1}^{m}p_i^2\ \#0.5\ \forall\ \ell$$

$$f_A=\frac{k}{m}-\frac{j}{m}$$

A very simple estimator. This estimator is also independent from f_A and need therefore no prior assumptions.

Let us study the weight $w_\ell=\left(1-\frac{2h_\ell-1}{h_\ell+(1-h_\ell)f_A}\right)$ of a homozygous locus according to

$h_\ell=\sum_{i-1}^{n}p_i^2$ and the prior on f_A.These weights are indeed functions of the parameters that we are trying to estimate. Their estimation needs therefore prior assumptions or iterative resolution. We can also remark that h_ℓ is the inverse of the effective number of alleles A_e at the locus (i.e the equivalent number of alleles when even frequencies; A_e=2 for two equiprobable alleles, A_e=n for n equiprobable alleles). The weight r_ℓ can easily be expressed in terms of A_e:

$$w_\ell=\left\{1-\frac{(2-A_e)}{[1+(A_e-1)]f_A}\right\}$$

The same argument at the allele level (not as before at the locus level) starting from the formulae just before (1) leads to similar results. In this case the weights w*i* take in account p*i* the allele frequency changing h*l* in p*i*.

Table 3 and Figure 2 shows that this weight increases as h_ℓ tends to zero and as f_A tends also to zero. This increase tends to be very drastic for h_ℓ being under 0.10 and f_A smaller than 0.05.

Table 3. r_ℓ *weight of a homozygote locus in estimation of* f *by MLE according to* h_ℓ *probability of AIS and the prior on* f.

$$w_\ell = \left(1 - \frac{2\,h_\ell - 1}{h_\ell + (1-h_\ell)\,f_A}\right) \qquad h_\ell = \sum_{i=1}^{n_\ell} p_i^2$$

	f_A						
h_ℓ	0	0.01	0.05	0.125	0.25	0.50	1
0.05	**19.000**	**16.126**	**10.231**	**6.333**	4.130	2.714	1.9
0.10	**9.000**	**8.339**	**6.517**	4.765	3.462	2.455	1.8
0.20	4.000	3.885	3.500	3.000	2.500	2.000	1.6
0.30	2.333	2.303	2.194	2.032	1.842	1.615	1.4
0.40	1.500	1.493	1.784	1.421	1.364	1.286	1.2
0.50	**1**	**1**	**1**	**1**	**1**	**1**	**1**
0.60	0.667	0.669	0.677	0.692	0.714	0.750	0.8
0.70	0.429	0.431	0.441	0.458	0.484	0.529	0.6
0.80	0.250	0.252	0.259	0.273	0.294	0.158	0.2
0.90	0.111	0.112	0.116	0.123	0.135	0.158	0.2
1	0	0	0	0	0	0	0

This over weighting of some homozygous loci favouring very polymorphic loci (or rare alleles) will make the estimation of f_A too much dependent of the situation of identity observed at few loci and the exact determination of alleles frequencies at such loci will be more difficult due to the low expected values. Contrary to general agreement I would therefore not recommend to use such loci. Biallelic loci with the value of h_ℓ not so far from 0.5 would in my opinion allow more precise estimations because they are independent of the prior on f_A and are allowing more precise estimations of alleles frequencies. Table 4 shows the variations in h_ℓ according to n the number of alleles and a frequency disequilibrium supposing a constant decrease of allele frequency from the most to the least frequent one. It can be observed that h_ℓ is minimum for evenness and is decreasing with the number of alleles. Near 0.5 values for h_ℓ are more easily obtained for bi allelic loci, multi allelic have to respect a constant decrease in alleles frequencies near 0.30 to satisfy to the condition. This observation is leading us to propose a kit of single nucleotide polymorphism (SNP) to study parentage and connected problems in horse populations.

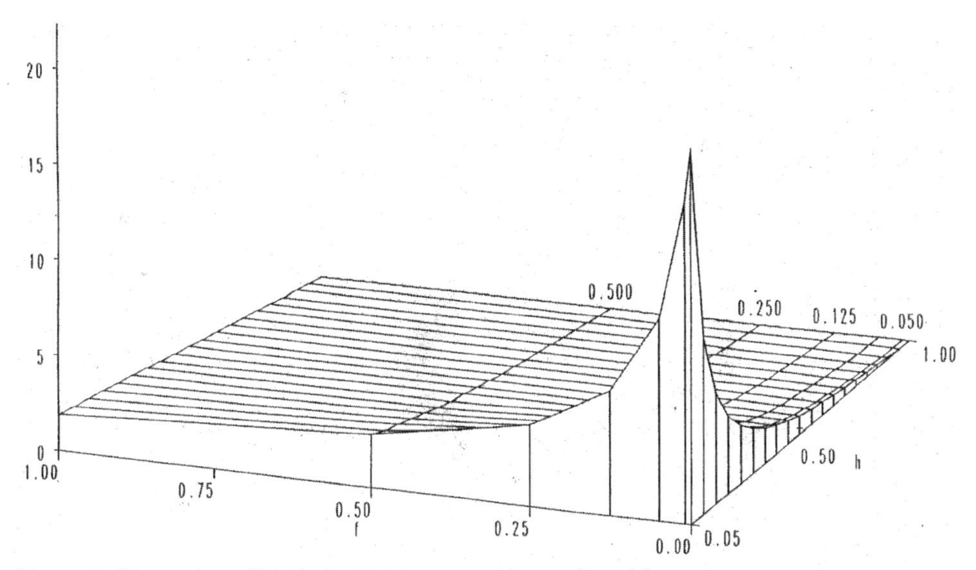

Figure 2. Illustration of Table 3: Weight r according to h and f.

Table 4. h_ℓ *probability of being alike in state according to the number of alleles n and a model supposing constant decrease of allele frequency from the most to the least frequent one.* $0 < a < 1$ *is the constant percentage of decrease.* $a=1$ *represent the even frequencies case.* $h_\ell = \sum_{i=1}^{n_\ell} p_i^2$.

a	n 2	3	4	5	10	20
0.1	0.835	0.820	0.818	0.818	0.818	0.818
0.2	0.722	0.677	0.669	0.667	0.667	0.667
0.3	0.645	**0.568**	**0.547**	**0.541**	**0.538**	**0.538**
0.4	0.592	0.487	0.451	0.437	0.429	0.429
0.5	**0.556**	0.429	0.378	0.355	0.334	0.333
0.6	**0.531**	0.388	0.324	0.292	0.253	0.250
0.7	**0.516**	0.361	0.288	0.248	0.187	0.177
0.8	**0.506**	0.344	0.265	0.219	0.138	0.114
0.9	**0.501**	0.336	0.253	0.204	0.109	0.067
1.0	**0.500**	0.333	0.250	0.200	0.100	0.050

Promoting the realisation of a kit of SNP

From the above studies it can be concluded that parentage analysis need a lot of markers to reach a reasonably good precision in practice. The problem to ascertain sire and dam of a foal is not so complicated and we have shown (Table 1) that 11 polymorphic microsatellites markers are sufficient to solve it properly. However the problem of remote parentage remains open and pedigree information is often not available to solve it. To help for the resolution of this dilemma we propose the realisation of a kit of SNP.

This kind of markers has the advantage of being easily revealed by DNA chips, being bi-allelic, co-dominant and null alleles free. This greatly simplify their management in terms of population genetics. Although not as discriminant as polymorphic loci, 5 to 10 SNP are considered equivalent from this standpoint to one microsatellite.

It is thought in addition that a SNP can be found in mammals every 500 to 1000 pairs of bases. Microsatellites are expected only every 25 to 100 kilo-bases. The screening of horse genome would be therefore much more precise with SNP than with microsatellites.

It is also known that mammal's genome is approximately constituted by 60 segments of 50 centimorgans. 60 independent markers at a bare minimum can therefore be expected and 120 at the maximum.

Conclusion

Due to their potential great number and their revelation facilities (positive or negative responses on DNA chips) allowing to squize sequencing for routine analysis, SNP markers allow to consider the tracing of parentage.

The realisation of a kit of several hundreds of SNPs would allow precise estimation of allele frequencies and a choice of 100-120 independent loci to trace the parentage as seen before. This could be a goal for at the end a better mastering the real parentage between individuals. For small populations the question of the evolution of inbreeding should also be better faced than actually by only taking pedigrees in account.

This new kit would also facilitate the comparisons of horse populations according to more precise genetic distances.

The realisation of such a tool is only a problem of engineering and financing not a question of know how. In my opinion from the solution of this political problem will depend the future of genomic in horse breeding. I treated here only one part of the whole problem. But this part appears sufficient to justify the approach.

Acknowledgements

We thank Louis Ollivier for helpful comments

References

Amigues, Y., J.C. Mériaux and M.Y. Boscher, 2000. Utilisation de marqueurs génétiques en sélection les activités de Labogéna. Inra Prod. Anim.,n° hors série "Génétique moléculaire : principes et applications aux populations animales",203-210.

Ayman, N. and R. Chakraborty, 1982. Evaluation of paternity-testing data from the joint distribution of paternity index and the rate of exclusion. Hereditas, 96, 49-54.

Binns, M.M., N.G. Holmes, A. Holliman and A.M. Scott, 1995. The identification of polymorphic microsatellite loci in the horse and their use in thoroughbred parentage testing British Veterinary Journal, 151, 9-15.

Breen, M., G. Lindgren, M.M. Binns, J. Norman, Z. Irvin, K. Bell, K. Sandberg and H. Ellegren, 1997. Genetical and physical assignments of equine microsatellites – First integration of anchored markers in horse genome mapping. Mamm. Genome, 8, 267-273.

Chakraborty, R., M. Shaw and W.J. Schull, 1974. Exclusion of paternity, the current state of the art. Am. J. Hum. Genet., 26, 477-488.

Cho, G.J. and B.W. Cho, 2004. Microsatellite DNA typing using 16 markers for parentage verification of the Korean native horse. Asian-Aust. J. Anim. Sci. 17(6) 750-754.
Cothran, E.G., J.W. Mac Cluer, L.R. Weitkamp, D.W. Pfenning and A.J. Boyce, 1984. Inbreeding and reproductive performance in standardbred horses. J. Heredity, 75, 220-224.
Cotterman, C.W., 1940. A calculus for statistico-genetics. PhD Thesis, University, Columbus, Ohio.
Cunningham, E.P., J.J. Dooley, R.K. Splan and D.G. Bradley, 2001. Microsatellite diversity, pedigree relatedness and the contributions of founder lineages to thoroughbred horses. Animal Genetics,32, 360-364.
Devlin, B., K. Roeder and N.C. Ellstrand, 1988. Fractional paternity assignment: theoretical development and comparison to other methods. Theor. Appl. Genet., 76, 369-380.
Dodds, K.G., M.L. Tate, J.C. Mc Evan and A.H. Crawford, 1996. Exclusion probabilities for pedigree testing farm animals Theor. Appl. Genet., 92, 966-975
Eding, H., 2002. Conservation of genetic diversity. PhD. Thesis 120p.
Eding, H. and T.H.E. Meuwissen, 2001. Marker based estimates of between and within population kinships for the conservation of genetic diversity. J. of Anim. Breed. Genet., 118, 141-159.
Ellegren, H., Johansson M., Sandberg K., Anderson L., 1992. Cloning of highly polymorpic microsatellites in the horse. Animal Genetics, 23, 133-142.
Gerber, S., S. Mariette, R. Streiff, C. Bodénès and A. Kremer, 2000. Comparison of microsatellites and amplified fragment lenght polymorphysm markers for parentage analysis Mol. Ecol., 9, 1037-1048.
Guérin, G., M. Bertaud and Y. Amigues, 1994. Characterization of seven new horse microsatellites: HMS1, HMS2, HMS3, HMS5, HMS6, HMS7 and HMS8. Animal Genetics, 25, 62.
Jacquard, A., 1972. Genetic information given by a relative. Biometrics, 28, 1101-1114.
Jamieson, A., St.C.S. Taylor, 1997. Comparisons of three probability formulae for parentage exclusion. Anim. Genet. 28, 397-400.
Jones, A., W.R. Ardren, 2003. Methods of parentage analysis in natural populations. Molecular Ecology, 12, 2511-2523.
Kavar, T., G. Brem, F. Habe and J. Sölkner, Dovc P. 2002. History of Lipizzan horse maternal lines revealed by mtDNA analysis. Genet. Sel. Evol. 34, 635-648.
Li, C.C. and D.G.Horvitz, 1953. Some methods of estimating the inbreeding coefficient. Am. J. Hum. Genet., 5, 107-117.
Li, C.C., D.E. Weeks and A. Chakravati, 1993.Similarity of DNA fingerprints due to chance and relatedness. Hum. Hered. 43, 45-52.
Lynch, M. and K. Ritland, 1999. Estimation of pairwise relatedness with molecular markers. Genetics, 152, 1753-1766.
Lynch, M., 1988. Estimation of relatedness by DNA fingerprinting. Mol. Biol. Evol., 5, 584-599.
Mac Cluer, J.W., A.J. Boyce, B. Dyke, L.R. Weitkamp, D.W. Pfenning and C.J. Parsons, 1983. Inbreeding and pedigree structure in Standard bred horses. J. Heredity, 74, 394-399.
Mahon, G.A.T. and E.P. Cunningham, 1982. Inbreeding and the inheritance of fertility in Thoroughbred mare. Livest. Prod. Sci., 9, 743-754.
Malécot, G., 1948. Les mathématiques de l'hérédité. Paris, Masson et Cie.64p.
Malécot, G. 1969. Consanguinité panmictique et consanguinité systématique (coefficients de Wright et de Malécot). Ann. Génét. Sél. Anim. 1, 237-242.
Marklund, S., H. Ellegren, S. Eriksson, K. Sandberg and L. Anderson, 1994. Parentage testing and linkage analysis in the horse using a set of highly polymorphic microsatellites. Anim. Genet., 25, 19-23.
Marshall, T.C., J. Slate, L.E.B. Kruuk and J.M. Pemberton, 1998. Statistical confidence for likelihood – based paternity inference in natural populations. Mol. Ecol., 7, 639-655.
Meagher, T., 1986. Analysis of paternity within a natural population of chromaelirum luteus I Identification of the most likely parents. Am. Nat., 128, 199-215.
Meagher, T.R. and E.A. Thompson, 1986. The relationship between single and parent pair genetic likelihoods in genealogy reconstruction. Theoretical Population Biology, 29, 87-107.
Meagher, T.R. and E.A. Thompson, 1987. Analysis of parentage for naturally established seedlings within a population of Chamaelirium luteum (liliaceae). Ecology, 68, 803-812.
Moureaux, S., E. Verrier, A. Ricard and J.C. Mériaux, 1996. Genetic varaibility within French race and riding horse breeds from genealogical data and blood marker polymorphisms. Genet. Sel. Evol., 28, 83-102.
Queller, D.C. and K.F. Goodnight, 1989. Estimating relatedness using genetic markers. Evolution 43,258-275.
Ritland, K., 1996. Estimators for pairwise relatedness and individual inbreeding coefficients. Genet. Res., 67, 175-186.
Robertson, A. and W.G. Hill, 1984. Deviation from Hardy Weinberg proportions: sampling variances and use in estimation of inbreeding coefficients 1984. Genetics, 107, 703-718.
San Cristobal, M. and C. Chevalet, 1997. Error tolerant parent identification from a finite set of individuals Genet. Res., 70, 53-62.

Selvin, S., 1980. Probability of non paternity determined by multiple allele co-dominant systems. Am. J. Hum. Genet., 32, 276-278.
Smouse, P.E. and R. Chakraborty, 1986. The use of restriction fragment length polymorphism in paternity analysis. Am. J. Hum. Genet., 38, 918-939.
Thompson, E.A. 1975. The estimation of pairwise relationships. Ann. Hum. Genet. Lond., 39, 173-188.
Thompson, E.A. 1976. Inference of genealogical structure. Social Sciences Information 15,477-526.
Thompson, E.A. and T.R. Meagher, 1987. Parental and sib likelihoods in genealogy reconstitution. Biometrics, 43, 585-600.
Van Haeringen, H., A.T. Bowling, M.L. Stott, J.A. Lenstra and K.A. Zwaagstra, 1994. A highly polymorphic horse microsatellite locus: VHL20. Anim. Genet., 25, 207.
Wright, S., 1978. Evolution and the Genetics of Populations, Vol 4, Variability within and among Natural Populations. Univ. of Chicago press, Chicago, USA.
Zechner, P., J. Sölkner, I. Bodo, T. Druml, R. Baumung, R. Achmann, E. Marti, F. Habe and G. Brem, 2002. Analysis of diversity and population structure in the lipizzan horse breed based on pedigree information. Livest. Prod. Sci. 77, 137-146.

Genetic distance as a tool in the conservation of rare horse breeds

E.G. Cothran[1] *and C. Luis*[2]

[1]*Department of Veterinary Science, University of Kentucky, Lexington, KY 40546, USA*
[2]*Universidade de Lisboa, Faculdade de Ciências, Departamento de Biologia Animal, Centro de Biologia Ambiental, 1749-016 Lisboa, Portugal*

Abstract

The use of genetic distance measures calculated from genetic marker data for making decisions regarding the conservation of rare breeds of horses was examined. A variety of genetic marker systems (blood groups, biochemical variation, microsatellites, and mtDNA sequence variation) were compared. Also, different types of distance measures and clustering techniques were compared. Sample data from 22 horse breeds were analysed using various methods and the results compared. Genetic distance is a useful tool in the analysis of genetic diversity and relationships among domestic horse breeds. However, it should be used in combination with all information about a rare breed to make a determination of whether or not the breed is worthy of conservation efforts.

Keywords: genetic distance, genetic variation, horse, conservation, rare breeds

It is increasingly clear that the diversity of domestic animal resources used in agriculture is declining just as is the diversity of species in nature. Because the genetic diversity that is being lost could have importance to future agricultural production, efforts are now under way, lead by the Food and Agriculture Organization of the United Nations (FAO), to understand the current genetic diversity of the worlds domestic animal resources (for example see Barker *et al.*, 1998). The horse is included in this effort. Of all the domestic animal species, the horse has perhaps the greatest diversity of uses and has had a tremendous impact on human civilization first as a food source then as a means of draft power, transportation and as a weapon in warfare. Horses still perform all of their historical functions in one part of the world or another.

Genotyping of genetic marker systems now is frequently used as a tool for conservation. Probably the most important use is in the assessment of genetic diversity (Laval *et al.*, 2000). Another use is the determination of resemblance or relationship between and among populations by calculation of genetic similarity or distance (similarity is usually the inverse of distance; Hedrick, 1975). Genetic distance also can be used to determine population structure and genetic distinctiveness of a population or breed (MacHugh *et al.*, 1998). Here we will report on several aspects of the use of genetic distance as it relates to the conservation of rare breeds of the horse. In particular we will focus on the interpretation of the results of distance analysis and we will not go into detail on the statistical aspects of the various distance measures or clustering techniques.

The genetic distance analyses covered here were of 22 domestic horse breeds. The analyses were limited to this relatively small number of breeds to simplify explanation of the results. The breeds represent a wide diversity of horse types and include rare breeds. Three different data sets were analyzed. The first was 7 blood group and 10 biochemical genetic loci analyzed by standard techniques (Cothran *et al.*, 1998; Sandberg & Cothran, 2000) hereafter referred to as protein loci. The second data set was based upon 15 microsatellite loci also tested by standard methods (Juras *et al.*, 2003). Both the protein loci and the microsatellite loci are routinely used for parentage verification. The third data set was based upon 288 bp sequences of the mitochondrial D-Loop as described by Luís *et al.* (2002a).

A large number of genetic similarity and distance measures have been developed and used to compare groups of organisms. The various measures often have different statistical properties and are based upon different assumptions about how the variation among groups arose. There also are measures that are designed for specific types of genetic variation such as microsatellites or DNA sequence variation. All genetic distance and similarity measures are used to evaluate the amount of variation shared among groups (breeds for the purposes of this paper). The measures convert a large array of frequency or sequence data into a single value. Although this will result in some loss of information the single value simplifies looking at patterns among groups. Despite the different mathematical and biological assumptions the various measures are based upon, in practice most measures are highly correlated (Hedrick, 1975).

Tables 1 and 2 give distances values based upon protein and microsatellite data, respectively, for the set of 22 horse breeds. Although it is readily apparent that the distance values vary, it is not easy to determine how well the different measures correlated within data types or if protein data show relationships that are the same as the microsatellite data. You can compare the matrices statistically by use of the Mantel test (Mantel, 1967). A general discussion of the Mantel test is given in Hubert (1987). We give two examples of matrix comparison here (tests were performed using the NTSYS-pc package version 1.80). The first is a comparison of Nei's (1972) D versus the chord distance (Dc, Cavalli-Sforza & Edwards, 1967) for the protein data. The matrix correlation is 0.936 (this is equal to the normalized Mantel statistic Z). The approximate Mantel t-test value is 5.395, which is highly statistically significant. A scatter diagram of the matrix comparison is given in Figure 1. The high correlation of the two measures indicates that the two distance measures give essentially the same result. The comparison of Nei's D calculated from protein data and from microsatellite data gives a correlation of 0.665 and a t-test value of 4.133 (Figure 2). This also is a significant correlation but indicates that the two different types of gene markers show less correlation, even though the same distance measure is used, than do two different distance measures based upon the same data set.

Even though the distance measure is a reduction in the data from the basic gene frequencies, it still is difficult to evaluate relationships within a distance matrix. To further reduce the data and help to visualize the relationships among groups shown by the distance measures, a tree diagram (dendrogram) is usually produced using some type of clustering procedure. This reduces the data to two-dimensions. It also is possible to produce three-dimensional diagrams by use of an ordination technique such as principle components analysis or multidimensional scaling, but that type of analysis will not be covered here. There are almost as many types of clustering techniques as there are distance coefficients. These include a variety of phenetic clustering and phylogenetic reconstruction techniques. Again, the different techniques have different mathematical and/or biological assumptions associated with them. Different clustering procedures can give trees with different topologies from the same distance matrix.

Table 1. Distance matrices calculated from 17 protein loci. Da (above diagonal) and Dc (below diagonal).

ANDALUSIAN	0	0.078	0.100	0.095	0.075	0.086	0.081	0.078	0.081	0.148	0.122	0.069	0.086	0.146	0.036	0.075	0.047	0.075	0.195	0.138	0.121	0.156
ARABIAN	0.049	0	0.072	0.100	0.089	0.112	0.080	0.091	0.064	0.158	0.143	0.073	0.106	0.091	0.076	0.066	0.075	0.049	0.196	0.098	0.145	0.083
AKHAL TEKE	0.063	0.045	0	0.099	0.088	0.126	0.074	0.090	0.090	0.142	0.141	0.076	0.088	0.115	0.098	0.075	0.077	0.089	0.157	0.110	0.142	0.118
BRAZILLIAN CRIOLLO	0.060	0.063	0.062	0	0.066	0.111	0.080	0.064	0.118	0.143	0.109	0.071	0.095	0.105	0.092	0.074	0.061	0.073	0.179	0.101	0.128	0.124
CHILEAN CRIOLLO	0.048	0.056	0.056	0.041	0	0.083	0.055	0.049	0.079	0.118	0.100	0.054	0.072	0.118	0.059	0.063	0.047	0.054	0.182	0.096	0.123	0.117
CHILOTE	0.054	0.070	0.079	0.070	0.052	0	0.097	0.077	0.104	0.139	0.117	0.067	0.121	0.148	0.081	0.070	0.084	0.095	0.186	0.167	0.141	0.175
CONNEMARA	0.051	0.051	0.047	0.050	0.035	0.061	0	0.056	0.079	0.118	0.083	0.050	0.077	0.093	0.075	0.064	0.050	0.048	0.200	0.096	0.097	0.114
CAMPOLINA	0.049	0.057	0.057	0.040	0.031	0.049	0.036	0	0.079	0.114	0.090	0.045	0.068	0.111	0.070	0.060	0.037	0.054	0.168	0.098	0.099	0.119
CASPIAN	0.051	0.040	0.057	0.074	0.050	0.066	0.050	0.050	0	0.140	0.134	0.074	0.091	0.122	0.069	0.065	0.055	0.072	0.190	0.113	0.140	0.121
DALES PONY	0.093	0.100	0.089	0.090	0.074	0.088	0.074	0.072	0.088	0	0.072	0.095	0.111	0.161	0.136	0.114	0.121	0.133	0.208	0.128	0.127	0.179
FELL PONY	0.077	0.090	0.089	0.069	0.063	0.074	0.052	0.057	0.084	0.045	0	0.077	0.114	0.165	0.108	0.093	0.092	0.099	0.227	0.109	0.113	0.161
GARRANO	0.044	0.046	0.048	0.045	0.034	0.042	0.031	0.028	0.047	0.060	0.048	0	0.064	0.105	0.055	0.052	0.053	0.046	0.183	0.103	0.091	0.112
HAFLINGER	0.054	0.067	0.056	0.060	0.046	0.076	0.049	0.043	0.057	0.070	0.071	0.040	0	0.147	0.095	0.074	0.071	0.085	0.181	0.088	0.074	0.156
HOLSTEINER	0.092	0.058	0.072	0.066	0.074	0.093	0.059	0.070	0.077	0.101	0.104	0.066	0.093	0	0.121	0.110	0.105	0.068	0.231	0.120	0.167	0.059
LUSITANO	0.023	0.048	0.062	0.058	0.037	0.051	0.047	0.044	0.043	0.086	0.068	0.035	0.060	0.076	0	0.061	0.049	0.057	0.183	0.124	0.121	0.110
PERUVIAN PASO	0.048	0.041	0.047	0.046	0.040	0.044	0.040	0.038	0.041	0.072	0.059	0.033	0.046	0.069	0.038	0	0.060	0.055	0.190	0.096	0.123	0.115
PANTANEIRO	0.030	0.047	0.048	0.038	0.030	0.053	0.032	0.023	0.035	0.076	0.058	0.033	0.045	0.066	0.031	0.038	0	0.049	0.182	0.106	0.105	0.099
QUARTER HORSE	0.047	0.031	0.056	0.046	0.034	0.060	0.030	0.034	0.045	0.084	0.062	0.029	0.053	0.043	0.036	0.035	0.031	0	0.211	0.070	0.106	0.052
SORRAIA	0.123	0.123	0.099	0.113	0.114	0.117	0.126	0.106	0.120	0.131	0.143	0.115	0.114	0.146	0.115	0.119	0.115	0.133	0	0.192	0.205	0.236
STANDARDBRED	0.087	0.062	0.069	0.064	0.060	0.105	0.060	0.062	0.071	0.081	0.068	0.065	0.056	0.075	0.078	0.060	0.067	0.044	0.121	0	0.116	0.114
SUFFOLK PUNCH	0.076	0.092	0.089	0.081	0.077	0.089	0.061	0.063	0.088	0.080	0.071	0.057	0.046	0.105	0.076	0.078	0.066	0.066	0.129	0.073	0	0.176
THOROUGHBRED	0.098	0.052	0.074	0.078	0.074	0.110	0.072	0.075	0.076	0.113	0.102	0.070	0.098	0.037	0.069	0.072	0.062	0.033	0.149	0.072	0.111	0

Table 2. Distance matrices calculated from 15 microsatellite loci. Da (below diagonal) and Fst (above diagonal).

ANDALUSIAN	0	0.103	0.100	0.092	0.100	0.087	0.091	0.090	0.086	0.169	0.124	0.071	0.167	0.152	0.060	0.099	0.092	0.062	0.229	0.091	0.102	0.090
ARABIAN	0.181	0	0.080	0.114	0.142	0.092	0.108	0.103	0.074	0.181	0.142	0.086	0.190	0.138	0.067	0.103	0.101	0.087	0.229	0.095	0.157	0.123
AKHAL TEKE	0.160	0.105	0	0.114	0.129	0.075	0.077	0.107	0.075	0.150	0.114	0.056	0.162	0.106	0.064	0.098	0.092	0.060	0.223	0.100	0.096	0.109
BRAZILLIAN CRIOLLO	0.153	0.198	0.180	0	0.077	0.057	0.080	0.057	0.076	0.119	0.108	0.059	0.145	0.137	0.093	0.065	0.072	0.061	0.242	0.081	0.119	0.112
CHILEAN CRIOLLO	0.174	0.219	0.203	0.117	0	0.087	0.090	0.095	0.085	0.133	0.118	0.081	0.145	0.159	0.111	0.087	0.100	0.086	0.249	0.105	0.128	0.122
CHILOTE	0.157	0.147	0.101	0.116	0.147	0	0.064	0.047	0.054	0.112	0.107	0.027	0.132	0.121	0.065	0.052	0.056	0.050	0.219	0.087	0.094	0.099
CONNEMARA	0.181	0.174	0.121	0.161	0.191	0.125	0	0.087	0.072	0.116	0.082	0.054	0.109	0.109	0.082	0.078	0.097	0.060	0.260	0.080	0.090	0.117
CAMPOLINA	0.150	0.182	0.170	0.113	0.167	0.103	0.185	0	0.069	0.126	0.114	0.050	0.135	0.174	0.081	0.059	0.075	0.068	0.196	0.098	0.124	0.132
CASPIAN	0.163	0.111	0.090	0.155	0.178	0.096	0.125	0.144	0	0.106	0.082	0.038	0.107	0.107	0.069	0.062	0.060	0.058	0.202	0.062	0.095	0.104
DALES PONY	0.266	0.286	0.223	0.240	0.245	0.196	0.192	0.228	0.194	0	0.062	0.084	0.140	0.199	0.159	0.112	0.130	0.125	0.303	0.145	0.120	0.186
FELL PONY	0.224	0.227	0.190	0.231	0.245	0.196	0.163	0.233	0.163	0.107	0	0.070	0.113	0.165	0.131	0.108	0.120	0.098	0.282	0.106	0.097	0.154
GARRANO	0.139	0.165	0.110	0.130	0.162	0.073	0.117	0.120	0.094	0.138	0.142	0	0.112	0.103	0.054	0.052	0.053	0.040	0.199	0.069	0.066	0.088
HAFLINGER	0.259	0.303	0.222	0.251	0.247	0.218	0.172	0.254	0.180	0.224	0.210	0.193	0	0.206	0.155	0.136	0.156	0.134	0.279	0.139	0.120	0.198
HOLSTEINER	0.230	0.185	0.148	0.224	0.254	0.177	0.165	0.277	0.173	0.313	0.284	0.181	0.296	0	0.129	0.148	0.129	0.101	0.314	0.119	0.131	0.086
LUSITANO	0.123	0.113	0.103	0.165	0.181	0.116	0.143	0.159	0.106	0.249	0.231	0.115	0.234	0.176	0	0.079	0.082	0.045	0.185	0.084	0.107	0.091
PERUVIAN PASO	0.163	0.182	0.159	0.135	0.148	0.103	0.173	0.131	0.138	0.217	0.220	0.146	0.248	0.247	0.145	0	0.061	0.061	0.213	0.086	0.118	0.121
PANTANEIRO	0.148	0.187	0.179	0.125	0.170	0.130	0.203	0.128	0.141	0.242	0.253	0.135	0.263	0.253	0.161	0.134	0	0.080	0.251	0.102	0.080	0.125
QUARTER HORSE	0.134	0.128	0.085	0.117	0.153	0.097	0.103	0.150	0.100	0.213	0.178	0.096	0.211	0.141	0.086	0.130	0.164	0	0.206	0.038	0.085	0.044
SORRAIA	0.340	0.308	0.327	0.376	0.349	0.321	0.418	0.305	0.288	0.430	0.426	0.319	0.378	0.469	0.253	0.303	0.366	0.312	0	0.244	0.263	0.246
STANDARDBRED	0.170	0.140	0.136	0.156	0.213	0.152	0.156	0.192	0.119	0.269	0.208	0.157	0.245	0.197	0.144	0.180	0.205	0.082	0.351	0	0.114	0.074
SUFFOLK PUNCH	0.153	0.238	0.150	0.193	0.228	0.144	0.148	0.192	0.148	0.178	0.177	0.102	0.164	0.201	0.151	0.214	0.147	0.145	0.381	0.195	0	0.126
THOROUGHBRED	0.171	0.170	0.139	0.171	0.213	0.156	0.189	0.218	0.169	0.312	0.282	0.160	0.316	0.133	0.155	0.200	0.229	0.073	0.357	0.119	0.216	0

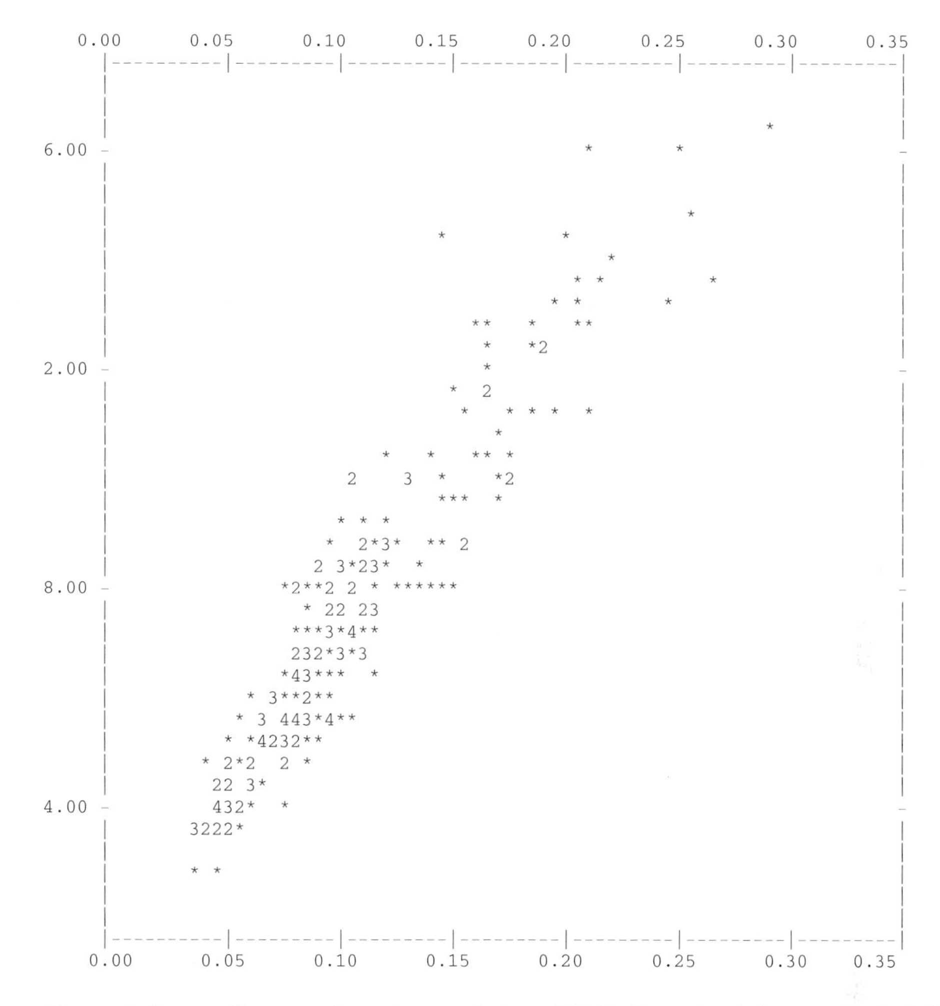

Figure 1. Scatter diagram of matrix correlation of Nei's D vs chord distance Dc both based upon 17 protein loci.

Figures 3 and 4 show Neighbor Joining (NJ; Saitou & Nei, 1987) dendrograms based upon protein data for 22 horse breeds and the Przewalski horse (used as the outgroup). Figure 3 is based upon the *Da* distance (Nei *et al.*, 1983) while Figure 4 is based upon *Dc* distance. The data sets were bootstrapped 100 times and bootstrap values are shown at the nodes of the trees. There are general similarities between the two trees but there are only four couplets that are the same (Thoroughbred/Holsteiner, Akhal Teke/Sorraia, Suffolk/Haflinger, and Fell Pony/Dales Pony) and only one cluster with more than two breeds that is the same in both trees (Thoroughbred/Holsteiner/Quarter Horse/Arabian). These are the clusters with the highest bootstrap values in both trees. The rank order of the bootstrap values is different for the branches between the two trees but mainly for the more distant branches.

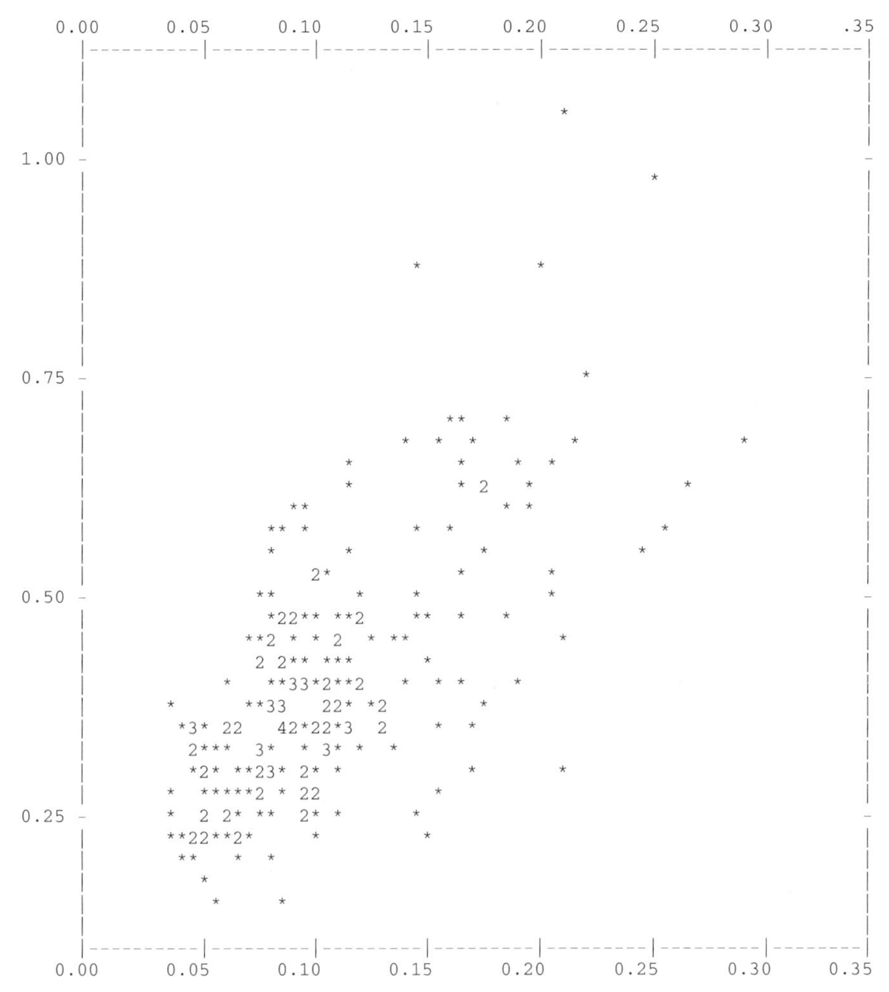

Figure 2. Scatter diagram of matrix correlation of Nei's D based upon 17 protein loci vs D, based upon 15 microsatellite loci.

Bootstrapping is used to give a measure of confidence in the way the tree reflects the total data in two dimensions. In general, the bootstrap values are low, especially at the nodes that connect the major groups. This is primarily due to the overall high degree of relationship among horse breeds. This causes inconsistent branching patterns at both the intermediate distances and at the outer branches, which leads to the low bootstrap values. However, this does not mean that the distance analysis and clustering cannot produce consistent trees that reflect true relationships. Although it is not extremely clear from the trees shown here, the major groupings of breeds shown do fit known relationships quite well. For example, for the most part Iberian type horses are grouped together as are the so called "cold blood" horse breeds, the draft and true pony breeds. If more breeds from each of the major groupings of horses were included in the analysis the major clusters would be more distinct (see Cothran *et al.*, 1998; Cothran *et al.*, 2001).

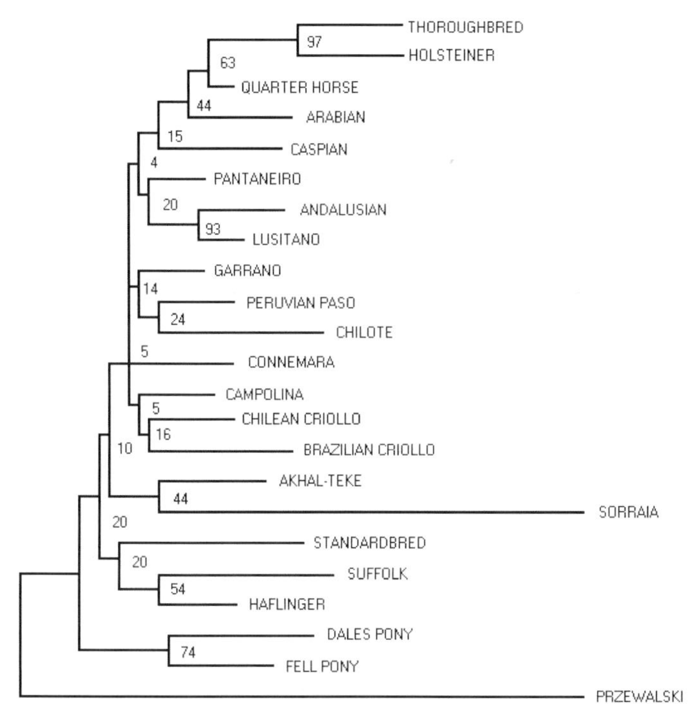

Figure 3. NJ clustering of Da distance based upon protein loci.

Figures 5 and 6 show NJ clustering of *Da* and *Fst* (Reynolds *et al*., 1987), respectively, based upon microsatellite data. For these trees, *Equus asinus*, the donkey, was used as the outgroup. Again, there is general similarity of the two trees, although there were only three couplets that were the same (Dales/Fell, Thoroughbred/Holsteiner, and Arabian/Akhal Teke). Also, bootstrap values are mostly low for the same reasons as indicated before. Again, despite the low bootstrap values, the trees do represent known relationships fairly well.

Comparison of Figures 4 and 7 shows how different clustering techniques can give different trees from the same distance matrix. In this case, *Dc* from protein data is summarized by the NJ method (Figure 4) and in Figure 7 by Restricted Maximum Likelihood (RML; Felsenstein, 1973). Again, there is generally a high degree of concordance between the two trees. Differences are mainly due to breeds that do not fit easily into any breed group or with other single breeds for a variety of reasons. We will go into this in more detail below. Except for these breeds, which include the Garrano, Connemara and Sorraia, there is fairly good agreement between these trees and, for the most part, the trees do reflect groups that are known to be related.

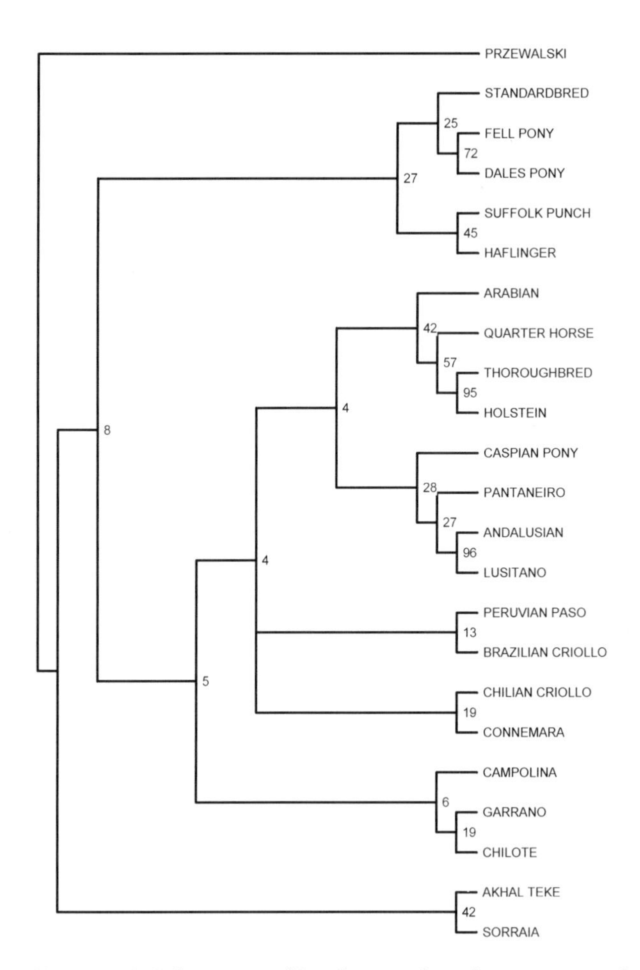

Figure 4. NJ clustering of Dc distance based upon protein loci.

Another type of genetic marker is mitochondrial DNA (mtDNA) sequence variation. The analysis of mtDNA variation has been tremendously useful in determining phylogenetic relationships of species and was used to clearly determine the origins of domestication of cattle (Loftus *et al*., 1994). However, as shown in Figure 8, mtDNA does not group breeds of horses into groups that fit expectations based upon recent history, nor does it match the groups shown in the protein and microsatellite analyses. This pattern has been interpreted to indicate a wide diversity in the geographic origins of horses in early domestication (Lister *et al*., 1998; Vilá *et al*., 2001; Jansen *et al*., 2002).

The analyses shown up to this point have looked at using genotyping data to compare populations or breeds. It also is possible to use this type of data to determine the population membership of an individual. Bjornstad & Roed (2001) have shown that the use of simple allele sharing statistics and maximum likelihood estimates, based upon allele frequencies, can achieve high power in the allocation of an individual to a breed for Norwegian horse breeds. However, Cañon *et al*. (2000) had lower success in correct breed assignments likely due to less genetic differentiation among the Spanish horse breeds they investigated. For the

Norwegian breeds a high probability of correct assignment was possible once more than twelve microsatellite loci were typed. This methodology could have use in breed conservation by determining which individuals, in a geographic region where breed designations are not well defined, make up a particular breeding group that could be considered as a unit for preservation. Also, it could be used to identify individuals that are members of a particular breed but have not been registered in a studbook. This would have value for a breed with a very small population size. However, this type of use of genotyping does require a good knowledge of the genetic structure of the populations being analyzed and there is always a possibility of error in breed assignment.

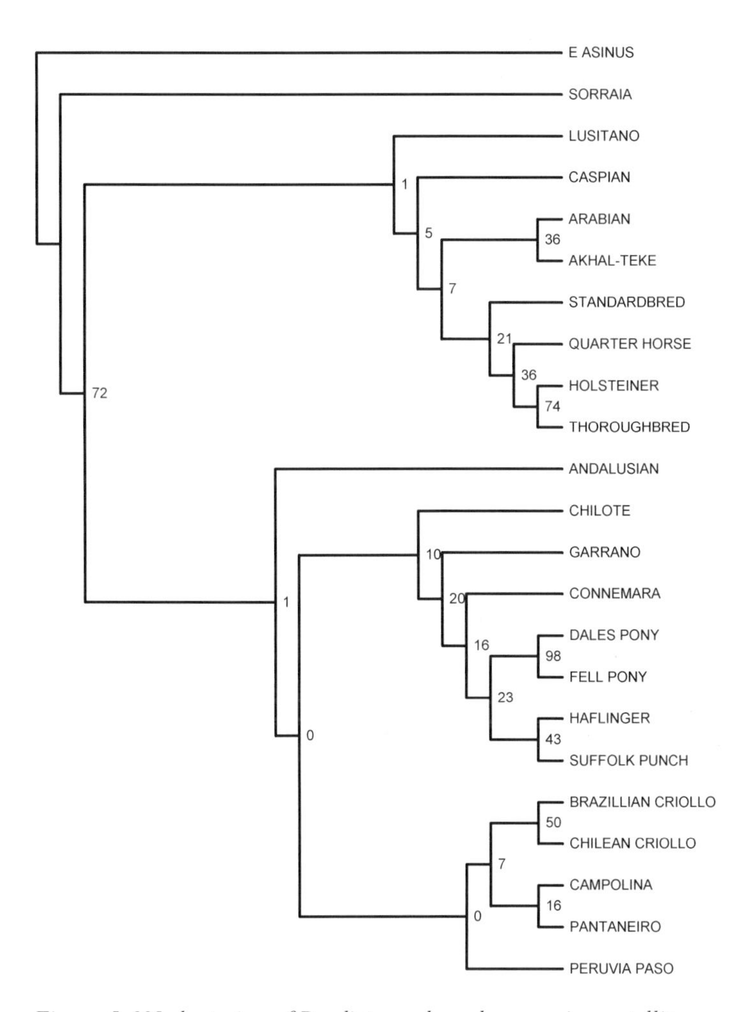

Figure 5. NJ clustering of Da distance based upon microsatellites.

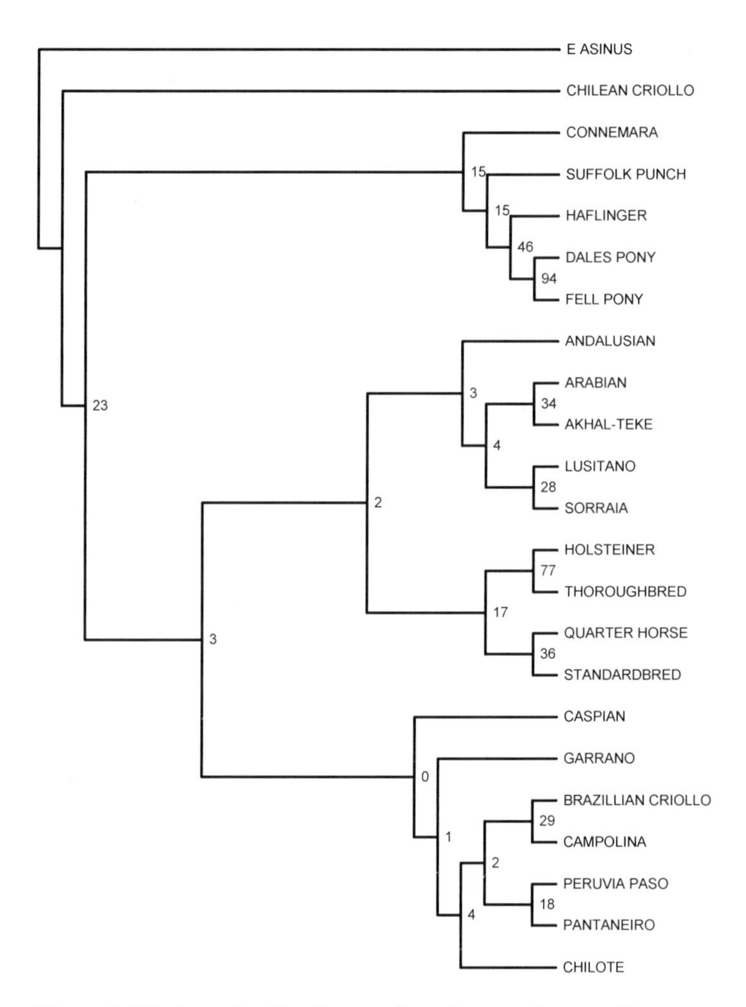

Figure 6. NJ clustering Fst distance based upon microsatellites.

The dendrograms shown here illustrate a number of points about genetic distance and clustering analysis that are extremely important to understand if these techniques are to be used for rare breed conservation planning. An important aspect of this type of analysis is that most of the clustering methods used are phylogenetic techniques that are designed to determine ancestor/descendant relationships based upon comparison with an outgroup. The outgroup is a sister group of the taxons being examined (in this case the horse breeds) which is used to determine which of the characters in the data are primitive to the groups and which are derived (Wiley, 1981). This type of analysis is not strictly appropriate to the analysis of breeds. Breeds do not evolve in a direct ancestor/descendent branching manner the way that species do. Because breeds are all members of a single species and are frequently formed by crossing two or more different breeds, the relationships among breeds of a species are more like a web than a tree. For this reason, a phenetic clustering method such as UPGMA, which only considers distance rather than assumptions about the character states, is probably more appropriate. However, in practice, a UPGMA tree of horse breed genetic distance such as shown in Figure 9 (based upon *Fst* distance and microsatellite data) does not give a tree that fits known relationships as well as the NJ or RML tree. The clusters in Figure 6 fit known relationships much better than those of Figure 9.

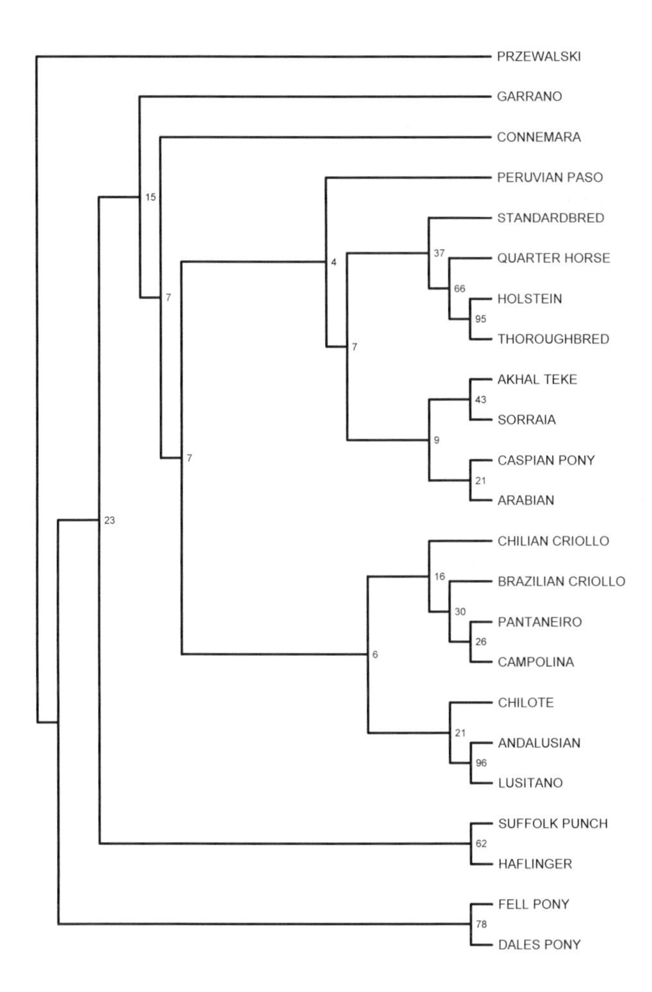

Figure 7. RML dendrogram of Dc distance based upon protein loci

It is very important in the interpretation of distance analysis that you know the breeds you are working with and the data. For example, the position of the Connemara varies among the trees. The Connemara is an Irish breed that is originally one of the native pony breeds of the British Isles. Thus, the expected position from that standpoint is that such as in Figures 5 or 6 where it is in the cluster with the Dales and Fell ponies and the Suffolk Punch, all British breeds. However, in Figures 3 and 7, the Connemara is in a much more divergent position and does not show any real breed group association. This is due to cross breeding of the Connemara to the Thoroughbred, Arabian and other breeds (Hendricks, 1995).

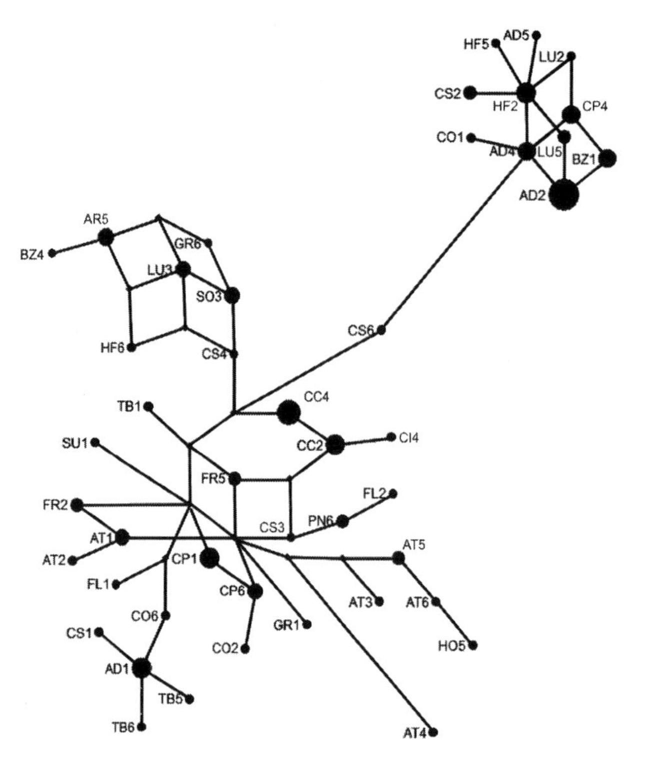

Figure 8. Reduced median network based upon 288 bp sequences of the mtDNA D-Loop region. Circles correspond to different haplotypes and are proportional to the number of individuals with the same haplotype.
BZ-Brazilian Criollo; AR-Arabian; LU-Lusitano; GR-Garrano; SO-Sorraia; HF-Haflinger; CS-Caspian; TB-Thoroughbred; CC-Chilean Criollo; SU-Suffolk Punch; FR-Friesian; CI-Chilote; FL-Fell Pony; PN-Pantaneiro; AT-Akhal-Teke; CP-Campolina; CO-Connemara; AD-Andalusian; HO-Holsteiner.

Knowledge of the data used in the distance analysis also is important for interpretation of results. Levels of genetic variability, for example, can have a major impact on genetic distance values. Figure 10 (based upon Table 3) shows the relationship of heterozygosity with *Da* distance for the breeds used in this study. There is a clear and statistically significant trend for *Da* to increase as heterozygosity decreases. This association also has been observed for breeds of chickens (Rosenberg *et al.*, 2001). The effect of variation on distance interpretation can be seen by the position of the Sorraia breed in the different trees. The Sorraia is a breed found in Portugal that may represent an ancestral type of Iberian horse (Andrade, 1926). It has extremely low variation, both in terms of allelic diversity and heterozygosity, due to a very small founder population size and a very small size of the current population (Luís *et al.*, 2002b; Oom & Cothran, 1994). In Figures 3 and 4 the Sorraia clusters with the Akhal Teke, a breed from the Steppes of Central Asia. In Figure 5, the Sorraia is the most divergent horse breed and is placed between the outgroup and all other breeds. In Figure 6, the Sorraia pairs with the Lusitano, another Portuguese breed and the one breed in this group that it is most closely related too. If one were unaware of the low variation of the Sorraia, the true genetic relationships of the breed could easily be misinterpreted. For example, if only Figure 5 were used the Sorraia could be considered as a very primitive breed. This may be true, but the primitive position in the tree is just as likely due to the low variability. Many of the oldest horse breeds do have low variability but it is not clear if this is a primitive condition or if it is due to small population size. Only the Arabian horse, of the oldest breeds examined to date, is not a rare or endangered breed.

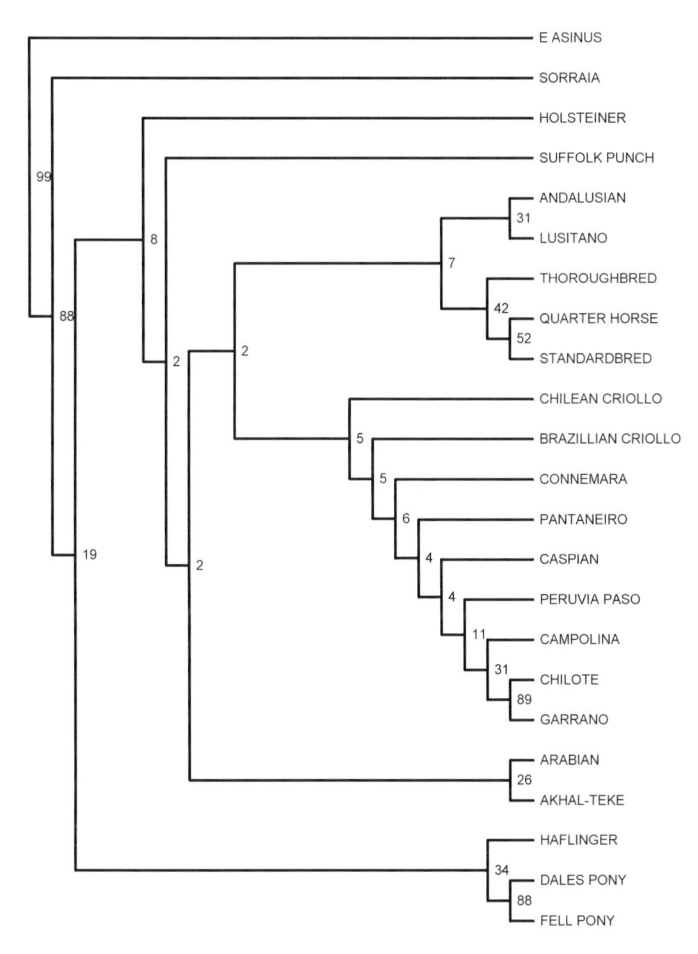

Figure 9. UPGMA clustering of Fst distance based upon microsatellites.

The Thoroughbred also has very low variation but consistently clusters where it would be expected in the trees shown. This is primarily due to relatively high number of alleles although allelic diversity (as measured by effective number of alleles, *Ae*) and heterozygosity are very low (Table 3). Rosenberg *et al.* (2001) also showed that allelic diversity was associated with genetic distance. In the case of the Thoroughbred, although it has low variation, it has been crossed into the Holsteiner and the Quarter Horse as well as a number of other breeds in this analysis. Thus, the Thoroughbred consistently clusters with the appropriate breeds even though only the Sorraia and Dales Pony have higher mean *Da* distance value when compared to the other breeds than does the Thoroughbred (Table 3).

Table 3. Hardy-Weinberg expected heterozygosity (He), effective number of alleles (Ae) and average Da distance for the 22 horse breeds, based upon protein data.

Breed	He	Ae	Da
Dales Pony	.382	2.026	.133
Arabian	.392	2.029	.097
Caspian	.404	2.066	.099
Thoroughbred	.319	1.842	.128
Quarter Horse	.439	2.585	.078
Holsteiner	.424	2.275	.124
Standardbred	.419	2.030	.113
Akhal Teke	.411	2.157	.103
Andalusian	.425	2.362	.099
Lusitano	.410	2.352	.089
Suffolk Punch	.466	2.282	.127
Haflinger	.458	2.534	.098
Chilean Criollo	.457	2.763	.085
Campolino	.457	2.589	.082
Peruvian Paso	.469	2.575	.084
Garrano	.447	2.361	.077
Brazilian Criollo	.463	2.569	.099
Fell Pony	.416	2.224	.117
Sorraia	.358	1.876	.194
Chilote	.449	2.392	.114
Pantaneiro	.439	2.534	.077
Connemara	.490	2.770	.084

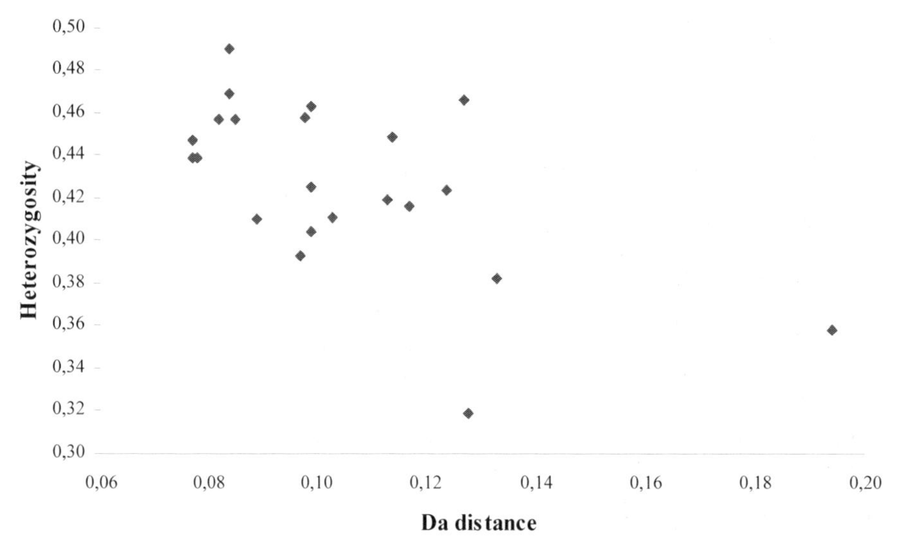

Figure 10. Plot of mean heterozygosity calculated from 17 protein loci and average Da distance for 22 horse breeds.

Of the 22 horse breeds used in the analyses reported here, seven could be considered as rare or endangered. These are the Akhal Teke, Caspian, Chilote, Dales Pony, Fell Pony, Sorraia and Suffolk Punch. What does the genetic distance analysis tell us about these breeds in terms of distinctiveness and relationship to other breeds?

First, in general, the cluster analyses of the distance measures places all the rare breeds within the major breed groups that they would be expected to be in, based upon their place of origin or known history, with the exception of the Sorraia. The Akhal Teke groups primarily with the Oriental type horses such as the Arab (Figures 5, 6 and 7) as would be expected based upon their origin on the Asian Steppes. The Caspian Pony, a breed of small horses from Iran, also fits within this group (Figures 3, 5 and 7). It should be noted that due to the small number of breeds examined here, major groups are not well defined but they are clearly apparent with a large number of breeds (see Cothran *et al.*, 1998). The Suffolk, Dales and Fell group together and with the Haflinger, which is the only other "cold blood" type horse in this analysis (Figures 3, 4, 5, 6 and 7). As noted above, the Connemara could be expected to fit within this group based upon origins but does not consistently do so due to recent history. The Chilote is a miniature horse breed from the island of Chiloe off the coast of Chile (Cothran *et al.*, 1993). It fits within the cluster of other South American and Iberian breeds. The Sorraia is an Iberian breed as well, but as discussed above, due to the low variation it does not fit consistently into any cluster.

The distinctiveness of these seven rare breeds is not easy to evaluate. All have mean *Da* values at or above the average for all 22 breeds analyzed here (Table 3). This suggests that they have distinctiveness at least as great as any of the other breeds. To some extent this is likely a result of reduced genetic diversity due to small population size, which is what defines these breeds as rare.

The only breeds analyzed here that are both rare and closely related (both genetically and geographically) are the Dales and Fell Pony breeds. The Dales is native to the eastern side of the Pennines of England while the Fell is found on the western side. The breeds probably share a common origin from a mixture of horses in the region in Roman times, but have slightly different histories of cross breeding in more recent times with the Dales being influenced by the Welsh Cob and Clydesdale to a greater degree than the Fell in the eighteenth and nineteenth centuries (Hendricks, 1995). The genetic distance analysis clearly shows the close relationship as the two breeds cluster together in all trees and the distance values between the two are consistently low. What the distance analysis does not show is which breed you might want to conserve if there were only resources to preserve one of them. Other physical and historical factors must be taken into account if such a hypothetical decision had to be made. If the decision involved preservation of two of the three rare British breeds analyzed here, the Suffolk Punch is clearly distinct from the Fell and Dales, both physically and genetically, so the decision would again come down to the two pony breeds. In physical appearance the two are quite similar with the Dales being slightly larger. The breeds have similar histories and both have been used for riding, packing and farm work (Hendricks, 1995). The only factor that might differentiate the two is that the Fell is known to have a lethal, immune deficiency gene in the population (Fell Pony Society, personal communication) that has not been reported from the Dales Pony. However, with small population sizes, a genetic defect could occur in any rare breed. The point is that genetic distance alone cannot be used to determine the uniqueness of a breed (although methods such as that of Weitzman (1992) or the marker-estimated kinship/core set method (see Mateus *et al.*, 2004) can be used for uniqueness estimate). All known information must go into decisions about whether a breed is worthy of conservation. Genetic distance analysis can be used as a tool to confirm suspected relationships or distinctiveness, but it is important that a full understanding of the data set analyzed and the history of the breeds be included in the interpretation of the results.

Genetic conservation of rare breeds of horses is a complex issue. In the developed countries horses are seldom used in agriculture and conservation of rare breeds is more a matter of emotional and historical factors than of economic ones. In those countries where horses are still significant agricultural animals they are usually not organized into distinct breeds. Regardless of the current use of horses, once a breed or geographic type is gone they are lost forever. It is important to conserve the different types of horses because preservation of the diversity of types of horses is preservation of a part of human culture.

Acknowledgement

C. Luís was supported by a PhD grant (SFRH/BD/3318/2000) from the Portuguese Foundation for Science and Technology (FCT/MCT).

References

Andrade, R. d', 1926. Apontamentos para um estudo sobre a origem e domesticação do cavalo na Península Ibérica Aproximações. Centro Tipográfico Colonial, Lisboa, 30 pp.

Barker, J.S.F., W.G. Hill, D. Bradley, M. Nei, R. Fries and R.K. Wayne, 1998. Measurement of domestic animal diversity (MoDAD): original working group report. Fao. Rome.

Bjornstad, G. and K.H. Roed, 2001. Breed determination and potential for breed allocation of horses assessed by microsatellites. Anim. Genet. 32, 55-65.

Canon, J., M.L. Checa, C. Carleos, J.L. Vega-Pla, M. Vallejo and S. Dunner, 2000. The genetic structure of Spanish Celtic horse breeds inferred from microsatellite data. Anim. Genet. 31, 39-48.

Cavalli-Sforza, L.L. and A.W.F. Edwards, 1967. Phylogenetic analysis: models and estimation procedures. Am. J. Hum. Genet. 19, 233-257.

Cothran, E.G., R. Mancilla, J. Oltra and M. Ortiz, 1993. Genetic analysis of the Chilote horse from the island of Chiloe-Chile. Arch. Med. Vet. 25, 137-146.

Cothran, E.G., S.A. Santos, M.C.M. Mazza, T.L. Lear and J.R.B. Sereno, 1998. Genetics of the Pantaneiro horse of the Pantanal region of Brazil. Genet. Mol. Biol. 21, 343-349.

Cothran, E.G., E. Van Dyk and F.J. Vander Mewre, 2001. Genetic variation in the feral horses of the Namib Desert, Namibia, Africa. J. S. Afr. Vet. Ass. 72, 18-22.

Felsenstein, J., 1973. Maximum likelihood estimation of evolutionary trees from continuous characters. Am. J. Hum. Genet. 25, 471-492.

Hedrick, P.W., 1975. Genetic similarity and distance: comments and comparisons. Evolution 29, 362-366.

Hendricks, B.L., 1995. International Encyclopedia of horse breeds. University of Oklahoma Press, Noman, 486pp.

Hubert, L.J., 1987. Assignment methods in combinatorial data analysis. Marcel Dekker. New York. 326pp.

Jansen, T., P. Forster, M.A. Levine, H. Oelke, M. Hurles, C. Renfrew, J. Weber and K. Olek, 2002. Mitochondrial DNA and the origins of the domestic horse. Proc. Nat. Acad. Sci., USA 99, 10905-10910.

Juras, R., E.G. Cothran and R. Klimas, 2003. Genetic analysis of three Lithuanian native horse breeds. Acta Agr. Scand., Sect. A, Animal Sci. 53, 180-185.

Laval, G., N. Iannuccelli, C. Legault, D. Milan, M.A.M. Groenen, E. Giuffra, L. Andersson, P.H. Nissen, C.B. Jorgensen, P. Beeckmann, H. Goldermann, J.L. Foulley, C. Chevalet and L. Ollivier, 2000. Genetic diversity in eleven European pig breeds. Genet. Sel. Evol. 32, 187-203.

Lister, A.M., M. Kadwell, L.M. Kaagan, W.C. Jordan, M.B. Richards and H.F. Stanley, 1998. Ancient and modern DNA in a study of horse domestication. Ancient Biomol. 2, 267-280.

Loftus, R.T., D.E. MacHugh, D.G. Bradley, P.M. Sharp and P. Cunningham, 1994. Evidence for two independent domestication of cattle. Proc. Nat. Acad. Sci., USA 91, 2757-2761.

Luís, C., C. Bastos Silveira, E.G. Cothran and M.M. Oom, 2002. Mitochondrial control region sequence variation between the two maternal lines of the Sorraia horse breed. Genet. Mol. Biol. 25, 309-311.

Luís, C., E.G. Cothran and M.M. Oom, 2002. Microsatellites in Portuguese autochthonous horse breeds: usefulness for parentage testing. Genet. Mol. Biol. 25, 131-134.

MacHugh, D.E., R.T. Loftus, P. Cunningham and D.G. Bradley, 1998. Genetic structure of seven European cattle breeds assessed using 20 microsatellite markers. Anim. Genet. 29, 333-340.

Mantel, N.A., 1967. The detection of disease clustering and a generalized regression approach. Cancer Res. 27, 209-220.
Mateus, J.C., H. Eding, M.C.T. Penedo and M.T. Rangel-Figueiredo, 2004. Contributions of Portuguese cattle breeds to genetic diversity using marker-estimated kinships. Anim. Genet. 35, 305-313.
Nei, M., 1972. Genetic distance between populations. Am. Nat. 106, 283-292.
Nei, M., F. Tajima and Y. Tateno, 1983. Accuracy of estimated phylogenetic trees from molecular data. J. Mol. Evol. 19, 153-170.
Oom, M.M. and E.G. Cothran, 1994. The genetic variation of an endangered breed: the Sorraia horse. Anim. Genet. 25 (suppl 2), 15.
Reynolds, J., B.S. Weir and C.C. Cockerham, 1983. Estimation of the coancestry coefficient: basis for a short-term genetic distance. Genetics 105, 767-779.
Rosenberg, N.A., T. Burke, K. Elo, M.W. Feldman, P.J. Freidlin, M.A.M. Groenen, J. Hillel, A. Maki-Tanila, M. Tixer-Biochard, A. Vignal, K. Wimmerg and S. Weigend, 2001. Emperical evaluation of genetic clustering methods using multilocus genotypes from 20 chicken breeds. Genetics 159, 699-713.
Saitou, N. and M. Nei, 1987. The neighbour-joining method: A new method for reconstructing phylogenetic trees. Mol. Biol. Evol. 4, 406-425.
Sandberg, K. and E.G. Cothran, 2000. Biochemical Genetics and Blood Groups. In: Bowling, A.T. and A. Ruvinsky, (editors) The Genetics of the Horse. CABI Publishing, Wallingford, United Kingdom: 85-108.
Vila, C., J.A. Leonard, A. Gotherstrom, S. Marklund, K. Sandberg, K. Liden, R.K. Wayne and H. Ellegren, 2001. Widespread origins of domestic horse lineages. Science 291, 474-477.
Weitzman, M.L., 1992. On diversity. Quart. J. Economics 107, 363-405.
Wiley, E.O., 1981. Phylogenetics. John Wiley and Sons, New York. 439pp.

Variation of mitochondrial DNA in Lipizzan horses

T. Kavar[1]*, F. Habe*[1]*, H. Sölkner*[2] *and P. Dovč*[1]

[1]*University of Ljubljana, Biotechnical Faculty, Department of Animal Science, Groblje 3, SI-1230 Domžale, Slovenia*
[2]*University of Agricultural Sciences, Department of Livestock Science, Gregor Mendel Strasse 33, 1180 Vienna, Austria*

Abstract

Mitochondrial DNA (mtDNA) represents an autonomous, from the nucleus separated genetic system of the cell with strictly maternal inheritance. Due to the high mutation rate within the control region, mtDNA is a suitable tool for tracing back the history of maternal lines in the pedigreed populations. Sequence analysis of mtDNA control region in Lipizzan horse, which represents the oldest European cultural horse breed, revealed 39 mtDNA haplotypes, exhibiting 0.14 – 3.5% sequence diversity within the breed. All Lipizzan haplotypes belong to four main equine mtDNA haplotype clusters (C1-C4). The haplotype frequency distribution in Lipizzan breed is quite unequal, reaching from 26% for the most common haplotype Capriola, which is present in 13 lines, to 0.2% for the rare haplotypes V, C and Z. Also the distribution of mtDNA haplotypes among Lipizzan studs is biased towards equal distribution of common haplotypes (Batosta) and occurrence of some rare haplotypes only in one or two studs. Comparison of pedigree data with molecular data identified several pedigree errors, which have occurred during the more than 400 years long history of the breed. We estimate that due to at least 25 historical pedigree errors, biological origin of about 10% of the Lipizzans is in disagreement with their pedigree data. In more detail the mtDNA haplotypes in the Slovene population of Lipizzan horses were analysed. Among 17 haplotypes, ten represent classical Lipizzan maternal lines, one Slovene maternal line Rebecca and six Lipican maternal lines of Croatian, Romanian and Hungarian origin. Based on sequence comparisons with a large set of D-loop sequences from other breeds, the origin of some Lipizzan mare family lines was elucidated.

Keywords: Lipizzan horse, mitochondrial DNA, pedigree, mare family line, founder mares

1. The Lipizzan breed

The history of the Lipizzan breed, which is the oldest European cultural horse breed, goes back to the year 1580, when the original stud at Lipica was established by the Habsburg Archduke Charles II. The primary goal of the stud was to supply the Habsburg court with riding and light carriage horses (Nürnberg, 1993). At the beginning, the horses from Lipica were known as "white horses of Karst origin", however, later the name Lipizzan horses was coined and widely used. The harsh limestone environment of Slovenian Karst at Lipica, from which the horse takes its name, favoured selection of horses with hard hooves, strong bones and contributed to the breed's soundness and longevity (Hortley 1994). (Figure 1.)

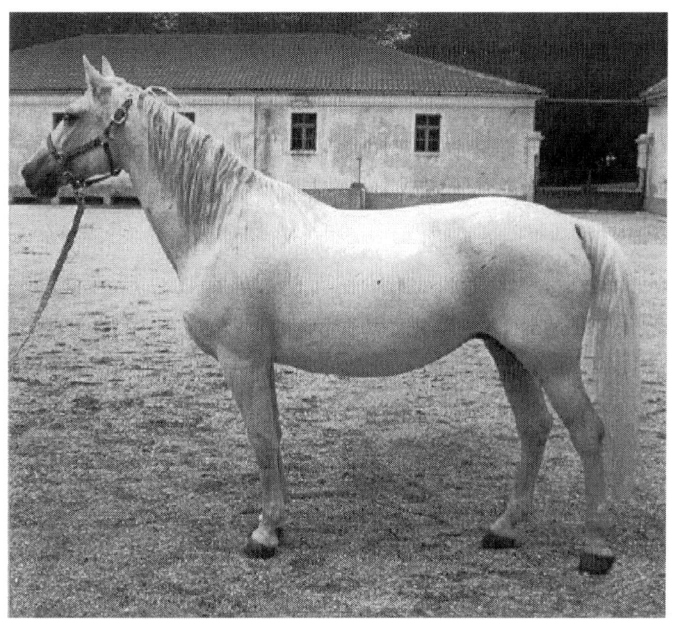

Figure 1. The historical stud of Lipica was established in 1580.

The basis of the breed formed the local Karst horses, horses of Spanish (Andalusians), Italian (Neapolitans, Lusitans) and Arabian (Arabs) origin (Nürnberg 1998). An important breeding practice was the exchange of breeding animals between studs within the Habsburg Empire (Lipica, Kladruby, Kopćany) and with the studs from abroad (Frideriksborg, Denmark). During the history of the breed, different stallion lines - the dynasties of very outstanding sires- were established. At present, there are six classical stallion lines of the Lipizzan breed: Maestoso, Favory, Conversano, Neapolitano, Pluto and Siglavy. As well as formation of stallion lines, establishing of maternal lines was inevitable for the development of the breed. Eighteen classical Lipizzan maternal lines were formed at the historical stud of Lipica. Eleven of them were established in the 18th century with mares from studs at Karst (Sardinia, Spadiglia, Argentina), Kladruby (Afrika, Almerina, Presciana, Englanderia, Europa), Kopćany (Stornella, Famosa) and Frideriksborg (Deflorata). During the 19th century imports of Arabs contributed essentially to the genetic base of the breed. Seven classical maternal lines of Arabian origin were established and four of them (Gidrane, Djebrin, Mercurio and Theodorosta) are still present at Lipica (Nürnberg, 1993). During the last century, the maternal line Thais (Rebecca), which originates from an imported founder mare of Arabian origin, was also established at Lipica (Dolenc, 1980).

The history of the breed is meticulously documented in the records on breeding practices and phenotypic characteristics of the horses. Almost complete pedigrees are available without gaps back to the early 1700 which makes the Lipizzan horse an unique and valuable object also for molecular genetic research. Today, the core of the Lipizzan breed is represented by eight state owned studs in the area of the former Austro-Hungarian Empire (Lipica, Piber, Monterotondo, Djakovo, Beclean, Fagaras, Topolćianky and Szilvasvarad). In addition, private breeders in more than 25 countries all over the world contribute to the preservation of the breed. The international umbrella organization of the breeders of Lipizzan horses is Lipizzan International Federation (LIF).

2. The equine mitochondrial DNA

Mitochondrial DNA represents an autonomous, from the nucleus separated genetic system of the cell with strictly maternal inheritance (Hutchinson *et al.*, 1974). Mammalian mitochondrial DNA is a circular molecule with the approximate length of 16.5kb. Apart from a short segment around the origin of replication, mammalian mtDNA is completely saturated with genes, all of which lack introns. The gene content and gene order are strongly conserved and include 22 tRNA genes, 2 rRNA genes and 13 protein coding regions, coding different subunits of the mitochondrial respiratory chain. The control region of the mammalian mtDNA functions as origin of replication for both strands and as promoter region with binding sites for the mitochondrial transcription factor. The control region is in the majority of mtDNA molecules in the mitochondrion characterized by the typical structure, called displacement loop (D-loop). Regarding the information content, mtDNA can be considered as haploid but regarding the copy number, each cell is polyploid, harbouring several tens to several hundreds of identical mtDNA molecules. Situation where the same cell contains two or even more different mtDNA types is called hateroplasmy and is considered rather as an exemption than as a rule.

Due to the relative high mutation rate, which is one order of magnitude higher than in the nuclear DNA, the mtDNA is often considered as a suitable molecule for measuring genetic distances between closely related species (Ishida *et al.*, 1995), within the species (Okumura *et al.*, 1996) and even within the breed (Bowling *et al.*, 1998). The extensive study of equine mtDNA was introduced by the sequence analysis of the D-loop region, the most variable part of the mtDNA (Ishida *et al.*, 1994) and by determination of the entire mtDNA sequence (Xu & Árnason, 1994). The evolutionary mutation rate within the non-coding sequence between the $tRNA^{Pro}$ gene and the central conserved sequence block (CSB) of the mitochondrial D-loop region in *Equidae* was estimated to be 2-4 x 10^{-8} per nucleotide site per year (Ishida *et al.*, 1995). Due to the high mutation rate in the D-loop region and strictly maternal mode of inheritance, became sequencing of the control region a widely used tool for tracing back the mtDNA sequence diversity among founder mares in pedigreed populations (Kavar *et al.*, 1999; Bowling *et al.*, 2000; Hill *et al.*, 2002; Kavar *et al.*, 2002).

Recently, the mtDNA was extensively used for the elucidation of the history of horse domestication. The mtDNA variability, found in the present horse populations, was used to estimate the minimal required variability in the ancient horse population, taking into account the time frame and mutation rate in the equine mtDNA. In addition to contemporary samples, archaeological samples, including mtDNA from Alaskan wild horse remains, preserved in the permafrost dating from 12.000 to 28.000 years ago (Vila *et al.*, 2001), were analysed. Extensive analysis of the large data set including 652 equine mtDNA D-loop sequences revealed 93 different mtDNA haplotypes, which clustered in 17 distinct phylogenetic clusters (Jansen *et al.*, 2002). Based on this data, the estimation was made, that at least 77 successfully breeding mares with unrelated mtDNA haplotypes had to be recruited from the wild during the domestication process. Since the mtDNA data do not show strong geographical signature (Lister *et al.*, 1998, Vila *et al.*, 2001), the most likely scenario of horse domestication includes a single domestication centre, from where the expansion of domesticated horses occurred relatively fast, covering the area from the antique Greece to China. The observed variation in mtDNA haplotypes could be explained by the local mares which were incorporated *en route*, forming the observed mtDNA clusters with the trace of the regional specificity (Jansen *et al.*, 2002).

3. Lipizzan mtDNA haplotypes

Sequence analysis of 212 Lipizzan horses revealed 37 distinct mtDNA haplotypes. Multiple alignment of these 37 Lipizzan haplotypes with the reference sequence (GenBank X79547, Xu and Arnason, 1994) showed, that the majority of the polymorphic sites (47) is located in the upstream part of the control region, whereas the downstream region is less variable (14 polymorphic sites). The Lipizzan haplotypes differ from each other in one to 24 sites, which generates sequence diversity in the range from 0,14 to 3,5%. Many haplotypes with sequence differences in the 5'-end had identical sequences in the 3'-end. The obtained Lipizzan haplotypes clustered in four haplogroups: C1, C2, C3 and C4. The bootstrap values were high for groups C2, C3 and C4 but slightly lower for the group C1. In spite of the lower bootstrap values in the C1 group, the integrity of the group is supported by the sequence identity in the downstream part of the D-loop. The four main groups could be further divided into subgroups. Within the C1 group haplotypes Slavina, Dubovina and X form one subgroup, whereas haplotypes F, G and Trompeta form the second subgroup. Splitting of C2 group into C2a and C2b as well as splitting of C3 group into C3a and C3b is even more obvious and is supported by high bootstrap values and almost identical sequences in the downstream region of the D-loop.

The comparison of the Lipizzan haplotypes with the haplotypes determined in other domestic horses showed clustering to the same four haplogroups (C1-C4) including several subgroups. Lipizzan haplotypes can be found in almost all subgroups with only a few exceptions. They are not present in the C3c subgroup, consisting of five haplotypes found in wild horses from the late Pleistocen from Alaska (Vila *et al.*, 2001). However, in the neighbour subgroup C3b the Lipizzan haplotype Thais can be found. In general, Lipizzan haplotypes are similar to the haplotypes found in other breeds; 15 of them (Allegra, Batosta, Capriola, Gaetana, Monteaura, Slavina, Wera, A, B, D, F, O, Q, S, V) are even identical with some haplotypes found in other horse breeds.

Multiple alignment of 37 distinct Lipizzan sequences with 146 equine control region sequences retrieved from the GenBank database revealed 116 distinct haplotypes and 89 haplotypes were observed only in one breed. On the other hand, some haplotypes (Gaetana, Monteaura, Allegra and O) were more frequent and were common in four to six different breeds. Usually, they are accompanied by haplotypes which differ from them by only one or two nucleotides. However, in some cases only the surrounding haplotypes or several closely related, more frequent haplotypes were observed.

From the total of 56 Lipizzan maternal lines analysed, in 38 lines only one haplotype was found, suggesting that there is no discrepancy among genetic and pedigree data. However, in 11 lines two haplotypes and in 7 lines three haplotypes were identified. Considering pedigree data we assume that at least 25 pedigree errors have occurred in the past. Because of the vertical transmission of errors through generations, we estimated that about 10% of present Lipizzans are in disagreement with their pedigree data.

The distribution of mtDNA haplotypes differs considerably among Lipizzan studs. Only the haplotype Batosta was present in all studs, but there were many haplotypes observed only in one or two studs. The haplotype frequency distribution in Lipizzan breed is quite unequal, reaching from 26% for the most common haplotype Capriola, which is present in 13 lines, to 0,2% for the rare haplotypes V, C and Z. The majority of haplotypes was present at low frequencies.

According to the sequences of the 5'-end (365 bp) of the control region, we can differentiate among 37 Lipizzan maternal lines. Sequences of the 3'-end of the control region did not contribute to additional differentiation. Therefore, for characterization of Lipizzan maternal lines, sequencing of the 5'-end of the control region is sufficient. The majority of 56 Lipizzan maternal lines could be characterized by distinct mtDNA haplotypes. The presence of 37 haplotypes reflects the broad genetic base of founder mares of Lipizzan maternal lines. High matrilineal diversity observed in Lipizzan horse breed was expected due to the independent development of Lipizzan maternal lines at several studs from founder mares originating from many different breeds, which were probably highly diverse. For example, in Arabian horses, which represent much larger population, only 29 distinct haplotypes were observed (Bowling *et al.*, 2000).

4. mtDNA haplotypes in the present Slovene Lipizzan population

The Slovene population of Lipizzan horses contains, according to the Slovene Lipizzan Studbook, 14 classical maternal lines, a new maternal line of Slovene origin Rebecca and two maternal lines of Croatian origin: Margit and Munja (Pangos, 1999). The stud at Lipica received in the course of exchange of breeding animals with the Hungarian stud Szilvasvarad also maternal line S14 Marquese (Table 1). Classical Lipizzan maternal lines were formed in Lipica from mares of Karst, Spanish, Italian and Arabic origin, prior to the World War II, whereas the newer Slovene maternal line Rebecca was formed after the war (Dolenc, 1980). The Croatian, Hungarian and Romanian maternal lines were formed mainly in smaller private or military studs in the former Habsburg monarchy (Ouhlela, 1996).

The information about the mare family lines could be obtained either from the pedigree data or by the molecular analysis of mtDNA. Due to maternal inheritance of mtDNA and low number of new mutations in the short period of time, we can expect that all animals, belonging to the same maternal line will have the same mtDNA haplotype. Therefore, we can assume that mtDNA haplotypes of founder mares were identical to the haplotypes, found in their descendants today. In cases, where different mtDNA haplotypes were found among the members of the same maternal line, pedigree errors can be assumed.

The molecular analysis of Slovene population of Lipizzan horses revealed 17 different haplotypes. All haplotypes with the exception of only two (Boka and Y) were already found in the previous study of the general population (Kavar *et al.*, 1999; Kavar *et al.*, 2002). Thirteen maternal lines were characterised by a single mtDNA haplotype. However, in three maternal lines (Gidrane, Deflorata and Munja) two or three mtDNA haplotypes were found (Table 1). This indicates that within these lines pedigree errors occured.

Because of sharing the haplotype Gaetana among the vast majority of animals from the mare family line Gidrane, Gaetana is most likely the characteristic haplotype for this mare family line. The same has been found also in other Lipizzan studs. Animals with the haplotype Y can be therefore considered as being misplaced within this line and should be put into a new maternal line. The same is true for the animals with the haplotype Capriola within this maternal line.

Table 1. Mitochondrial DNA haplotypes by mare family line. Column A – Lipizzan mare families in Slovenia, including place of birth of founder mares. Column B – haplotypes of Slovene Lipizzans. Column C – Haplotype distribution in Lipizzan population (Kavar et al., *2002).*

A Founder mare	B Haplotype	C Haplotype distribution
Classical mare families		
SARDINIA Lipica (SI)	Betalka	Capriola Betalka Monteaura
SPADIGLA Lipica (SI)	Monteaura	Monteaura Batosta Dubovina
ARGENTINA Lipica (SI)	Capriola	Capriola X
AFRICA Kladruby (Cz)	Batosta, Boka	Batosta Monteaura
ALMERINA Kladruby (Cz)	Slavina	Slavina Allegra
PRESCIANA Kladruby (Cz)	Capriola	Capriola Allegra Slavina
ENGLANDERIA Kladruby (Cz)	Allegra	Allegra
EUROPA Kladruby (Cz)	Trompeta	Trompeta
STORNELLA Kopćany (Sk)	Allegra	Capriola Allegra
DEFLORATA Frederiksborg (Dn)	Capriola, Betalka Gaetana	Capriola Allegra
GIDRANE	Gaetana, Y, Capriola	Gaetana
DJEBRIN Radautz (Ro)	Dubovina	Dubovina
MERCURIO Radautz (Ro)	Gratiosa	Gratiosa
THEODOROSTA Radautz (Ro)	Wera	Wera Allegra U
New Slovenian mare family		
REBECCA Vrbik (Hr)	Thais	Thais
Croatian mare families		
MARGIT Terezovac (Hr)	C	D
MUNJA Đakovo (Hr)	Gaetana, Strana	Gaetana Strana Slavina
Hungarian mare family		
S14 Marquese Mezohegjes (H)	M	M

In the maternal line Deflorata is the typical haplotype Capriola, therefore animals with other haplotypes do not belong to this line. In case of animals with the haplotype Betalka, the mistake was probably made in the studbook. Animals with the haplotype Betalka belong, according to the pedigree data, to the classical line Capriola and not to the line Deflorata. This is supported also by genetic data. For the maternal line Capriola is typical haplotype Betalka. We suppose that the mistake in the studbook was made due to many similar names, which appear in the lines Capriola and Deflorata.

The third example of disagreement between genetic and studbook data was found in the maternal line Munja, where haplotypes Strana and Gaetana were found. Since haplotype Gaetana is characteristic for the maternal line Gidrane, the haplotype Strana could be the correct haplotype for the maternal line Munja, especially because of the fact that haplotype Strana was not found in any other maternal line.

In addition, there were observed three new discrepancies between pedigree and genetic data in the Slovene population according to the distribution of mtDNA haplotypes in mare family lines in other countries. For the mare family line Sardinia is in the Slovene population the characteristic haplotype Betalka, but in other countries the prevalent haplotype is Capriola. Both haplotypes belong to the haplotypes, characteristic for classical Lipizzan mare family lines. Within the mare family line Argentina in Slovenian population was found only the prevalent haplotype Capriola. However, for the animals belonging to the mare family line Argentina from the Italian stud Monterotondo, the typical haplotype is X, which is not present at all in Slovenia. In the mare family line Europa was in Slovenia found only haplotype Trompeta, but in other countries the haplotype U. We assume that the frequent use of the name Trompeta in different Lipizzan lines caused this error. The haplotype U belongs to the classical haplotypes, whereas haplotype Trompeta probably belongs to a new mare family line Triglava with the founder mare born in Lipica in 1916. Mare family line Margit is an example for possible fixation of heteroplasmy. In this line haplotypes C and D, which differ only by one nucleotide, were found. Therefore the presence of two closely related haplotypes in this mare family line might be either a consequence of an error or fixation of two almost identical haplotypes, originating from the heteroplasmy.

5. The origin of Lipizzan haplotypes

Lipizzan mtDNA haplotypes cluster into four main haplotype groups: C1, C2, C3 and C4. Haplotypes within each cluster are characterised by a number of joint mutations. Haplotypes from the group C4 share for instance mutations at positions 15494, 15496, 15534, 15603, 15635, 16407 and 16563a, which once occurred and underwent fixation in the common ancestors of maternal lines belonging to the C4 group.

General comparison of Lipizzan mtDNA haplotypes with haplotypes present in other horse breeds revealed high degree of similarity, some haplotypes found in the Lipizzan breed and in the other breeds were even identical. These common ancestors of domestic horse were probably domesticated in the period around 6000 – 4000 years ago (Clutton-Brock, 1999). The genetic data show that there were a large number of wild females, belonging to different populations, integrated into the domesticated populations, bringing new mtDNA haplotypes to the domesticated population (Jansen *et al.*, 2002).

Due to the numerous migrations of horse populations in the past, it is relatively difficult to establish significant relationship between certain mtDNA haplotypes and different phenotypic groups (ponies, oriental horses, heavy drought horses etc.). Normally, all main haplotype groups (C1 – C4) are present in all breeds, also in the Lipizzan breed (Figure 2). Until recently, it was assumed, that all domestic horses originate from the same large population, which contained haplotypes from all major groups (Lister *et al.*, 1998). Further assumption was that different phenotypic groups appeared later, as a consequence of natural and artificial selection (Clutton-Brock, 1999). However, the recent results showed that there is at least a weak relationship between the mtDNA haplotypes and different phenotypic groups or geographical origin of the breeds.

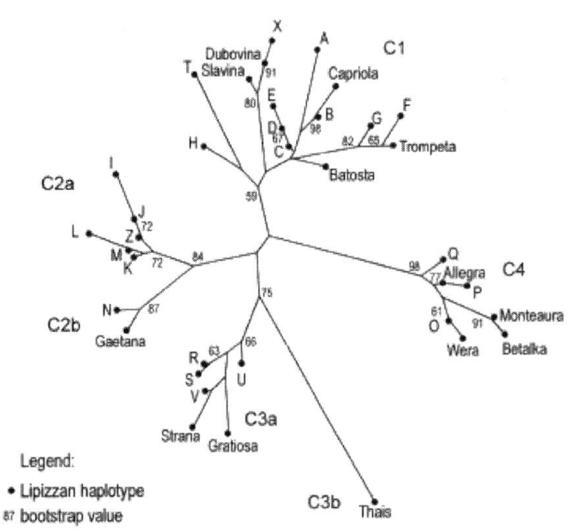

Figure 2. Relationship among 37 Lipizzan mtDNA haplotypes presented by the NJ tree. Bootstrap values higher than 59 were enetered into the tree. Haplotypes were clustered into four main groups (C1-C4) and into the C2a, C2b, C3a and C3B subgroups (from Kavar et al., *2002).*

According to that the C3a group of mtDNA haplotypes (Figure 3) should be characteristic mainly for the horses from Central Europe, British islands, Scandinavia and Iceland: Exmoor, Fjord, Iceland and Scottish highland ponies (Jansen *et al.*, 2002). Into the same group cluster also two Lipizzan haplotypes of Slovene origin: haplotype Strana, which is typical for the Croatian maternal line Munja and haplotype Gratiosa, typical for the maternal line Mercurio of Arabic origin. According to Jansen *et al.*, (2002), this group is called C1 and the group, mentioned in the next paragraph is called D1.

Due to the fact that during formation of the Lipizzan breed also Spanish horses were involved, finding that for the Iberian horses (Andalusians, Lusitans) and north African horses (Barbs) the characteristic haplotype group is C4, especially haplotypes Allegra and Monteaura, is of great interest (Jansen *et al.*, 2002). Both are also present in the Lipizzans in Slovenia. The haplotype Allegra is typical for five maternal lines, among others also for classical lines Englanderia and Stornella, which both originate from the Czech stud in Kladruby. This is not surprising, because horses of Spanish origin played an important role in this stud. The haplotype Monteaura was also found in the Karst maternal line Spadiglia. This could mean, that Spadiglia originates from Spanish horses, which were imported from Spain in the 16th,

17th or 18th century. The other possibility would be that haplotype Monteaura originates from horses, which were originally domesticated in Northern Africa, but arrived to the Karst area much earlier, possibly some thousands of years ago. Haplotype Monteaura belongs namely to the haplotypes, which are widely spread among domestic horses. There are at least 17 such common haplotypes (Jansen *et al.*, 2002). From the haplotypes found in the Lipizzan breed (Figure 4) belong to this group also haplotypes Gaetana, Allegra, Capriola and Dubovina. Because these haplotypes can be found in different breeds, we believe that they were already present at the very early stage of domestication. These haplotypes represent the group of older haplotypes, from which, during the history of domestication, more recent haplotypes were derived by accumulation of mutations. These derived haplotypes tend therefore to be present only in a smaller number of breeds. Two Lipizzan haplotypes, Betalka and X, which were derived from the haplotypes Monteaura and Dubovina, respectively, are examples of such younger, less common haplotypes. Haplotype Betalka seems to be present only in the Lipizzan breed, whereas the haplotype X was found also in the horses of Spanish origin (Mirol *et al.*, 2002). Such rare haplotypes will most likely be of great importance for tracing past migrations and relationships between breeds.

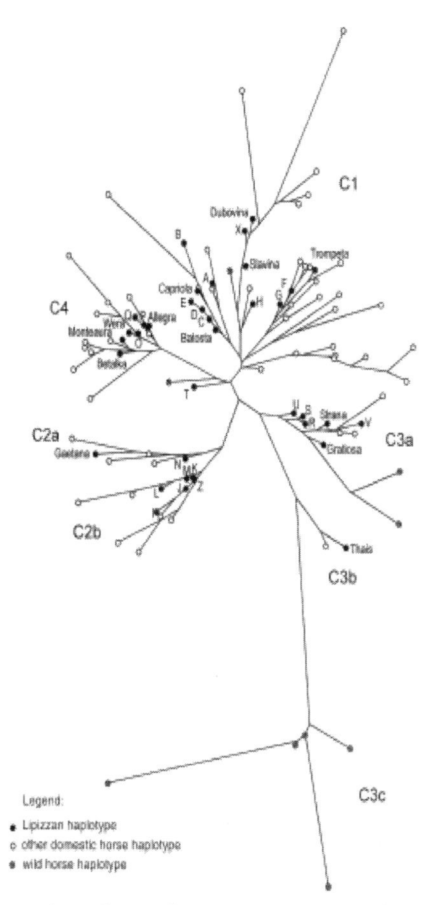

Figure 3. Relationship among Lipizzan haplotypes and some other domestic and wild horse haplotypes, represented by the NJ tree (from Kavar et al., 2002).

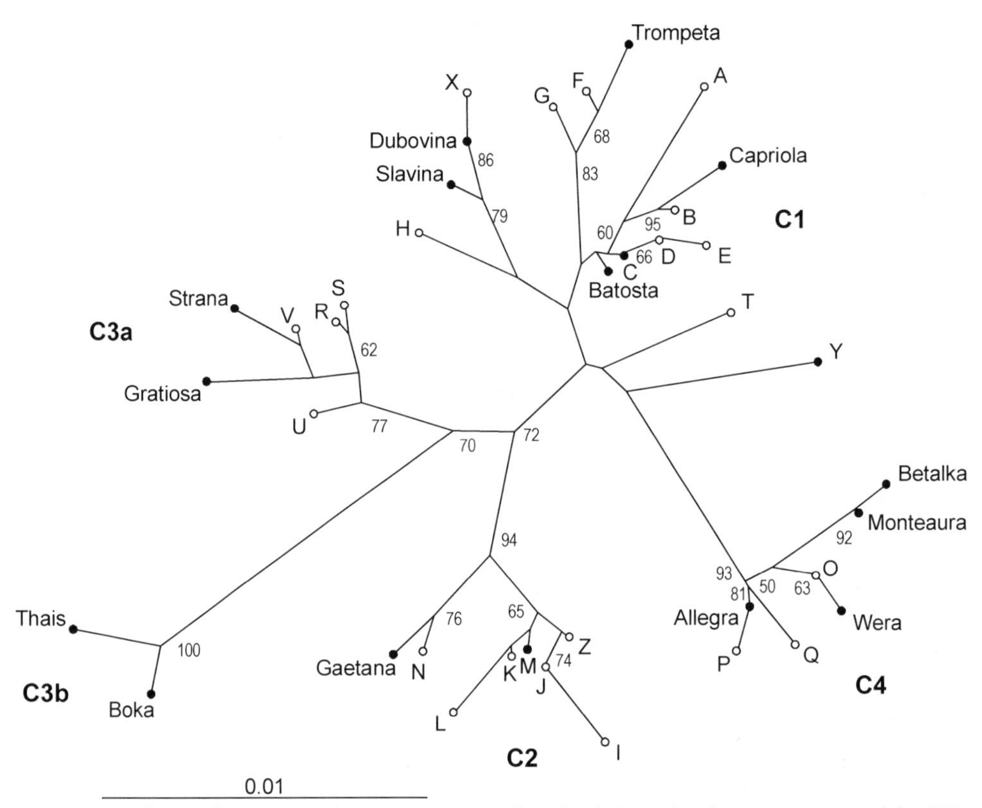

Figure 4. Relationship among 39 Lipizzan mitochondrial DNA haplotypes presented by NJ tree. Circles representing 17 haplotypes of Slovenian Lipizzans are in black (from Kavar et al., 2004).

Several connections between certain haplotypes and breeds from which different Lipizzan maternal lines originate were found. Interestingly, the most common haplotype among Arab horses, registered in the USA, was the haplotype which we called Gaetana in the Lipizzan breed (Bowling *et al.*, 2000). This haplotype is characteristic for Lipizzan maternal line of Arabian origin – Gidrane (Table 1). According to the pedigree data, the founder of this line was full blood Arabian mare OX Gidrane, which explains the connection with the Lipizzan breed. The presence of haplotypes Batosta and Slavina in the Kladruber horse breed and at the same time in the classical Lipizzan lines Africa and Almerina is also pointing out the connection between these two breeds, especially because both haplotypes were only found in the Kladruber and Lipizzan breed.

On the other side, we can only guess about the origin of the most common haplotype in the Lipizzan breed, Capriola, which belongs to the group of well spread haplotypes and can be found in three Lipizzan maternal lines (Argentina, Deflorata and Presciana) as well as in many other breeds (Connemara ponies, Trakeners, Fjord ponies, Dülmener horses, Holsteins, Arabs and Barbs).

In general, presented results support the assumption that there was considerable exchange of genetic material between breeds. The large genetic variability, present in the horse mtDNA, could be either the consequence of domestication from a large, heterogeneous population, or the consequence of multiple *en route* integrations of wild mares with different mtDNA haplotypes, to domestic horse populations during expansion of domestic horse across the Eurasian continent. The mtDNA can be successfully used for the reconstruction of the history of maternal lines within the breed, especially in situations, where less common haplotypes occur.

References

Bowling A.T., A. Del Valle and M. Bowling, 1998. Verification of horse maternal lineage based on derived mitochondrial DNA sequence. Journal of Animal Breeding and Genetics 115, 351-6.

Bowling, A.T., A. Del Valle and M. Bowling, 2000. A pedigree-based study of mitochondrial D-loop DNA sequence variation among Arabian horses. Anim. Genet., 31 (1), 1-7.

Clutton-Brock, J., 1999. A natural history of domesticated mammals, 2nd edn., Cambridge, New York, Melbourne, Cambridge University Press, 238 p.

Dolenc, M., 1980. Lipica. Ljubljana, Mladinska knjiga, 96 p.

Hill, E.W., D.G. Bradley, M. Al-Barody,O. Ertugrul, R.K. Splan, I. Zakharov and E.P. Cunningham, 2002. History and integrity of thoroughbred dam lines revealed in equine mtDNA variation. Animal Genetics, 33, 287-294.

Hortley Edwards, E., 1994. The encyclopedia of the horse, Dorling Kinderley Limited, London, p.110 – 111.

Hutchinson, C.A., J.E. Newbold, S.S. Potter and M. Hall Edgell, 1974. Maternal inheritance of mammalian mitochondrial DNA. Nature 251, 536-8.

Ishida, N., T. Hasegawa, K. Takeda, M. Sakagami, A. Onishi, S. Inumaru, M. Komatsu and H. Mukojama, 1994. Polymorphic sequence in the D-loop region of equine mitochondrial DNA. Animal Genetics 25, 215-21.

Ishida, N., T. Oyunsuren, S. Mashima, H. Mukoyama and N. Saitou, 1995. Mitochondrial DNA Sequences of Various Species of the Genus Equus with Special Reference to the Phylogenetic Relationship Between Przewalskii's Wild Horse and Domestic Horse. Journal of Molecular Evolution 41. 180-8.

Jansen, T., P. Forster, M.A. Levine, H. Oelke, M. Hurles, C. Renfrew, J. Weber and K. Olek, 2002. Mitochondrial DNA and the origins of the domestic horse. Proc. Natl. Acad. Sci. USA, 99 (16) 10905-10910.

Kavar, T., G. Brem, F. Habe, J. Sölkner and P. Dovč, 2002. History of Lipizzan horse maternal lines as revealed by mtDNA analysis. Genet. Sel. Evol. 34, 635-548.

Kavar, T., F. Habe, G. Brem and P. Dovč, 1999. Mitochondrial D-loop sequence variation among the 16 maternal lines of the Lipizzan horse breed. Anim. Genet. 30, 423-430.

Lister, A.M., M. Kadwell, L.M. Kaagan, W.C. Jordan, M.B. Richards and H.E. Stanley, 1998. Ancient and modern DNA in a study of horse domestication. Ancient Biomolecules, 2, 267-280.

Mirol, P.M., P. Peral García, J.L. Vega-Pla and F.N. Dulout, 2002. Phylogenetic relationship of Argentinean Creole horses and other South American and Spanish breeds inferred from mitochondrial DNA sequences. Anim. Genet., 33, 356-363.

Nürenberg H., 1993. Der Lipizzaner: mit einem Anhang über den Kladruber. Westarp Wissenschaften, Magdeburg, 250p.

Nürenberg H., 1998. Auf den Spuren der Lipizzaner. Olms Presse, Hildesheim, Zürich, New York, p. 20-41.

Okumura N., N. Ishiguro, M. Nakano and M. Sahara, 1996. Intra - and interbreed genetic variations of mitochondrial DNA major non-coding regions in Japanese native dog breeds (*Canis familiaris*). Animal Genetics 27, 397-405.

Ouhlela, J.,1996. Züchterische Standards in der Lipizzanerpferde-population. Habilitationsarbeit Brno - Piber, Fachtierarzt für Pferde und Tierzucht, 120 p.

Pangos, J., 1999. Rodovna knjiga lipicancev slovenske reje. Lipica, Kobilarna Lipica, 254 p.

Vila, C., J.A. Leonard, A. Gotherstrom, S. Marklund, K. Sandberg, K. Liden, R.K. Wayne and H. Ellegren, 2001.Widespread origins of domestic horse lineages. Science, 291, 474-477.

Xu, X. and U. Arnason, 1994. The complete mitochondrial DNA sequence of the horse, *Equus caballus*: extensive heteroplasmy of the control region. Gene, 148, 357-362.

Analysis of inbreeding in the genetic resource of the „Old Kladrub horse" in the period from 1993 to 2003

V. Jakubec[1], *J. Volenec*[2], *I. Majzlik*[1] *and W. Schlote*[3]

[1]*Faculty of Agronomy, Czech University of Agriculture, 165 21, Prague, Czech Republic*
[2]*National Stud at Kladruby, Kladruby nad Labem, Czech Republic*
[3]*Faculty of Agriculture and Horticulture, Humboldt University of Berlin, Germany*

Abstract

The Old Kladrub horse, which was established by the end of the 18th and at the beginning of the 19th century is the most important genetic resource in the Czech Republic. The structure of the breed in 2003 was: 39 stallions, 350 mares, effective population size (N_e) 140. The breed was closed against immigration in 1992 and since that time circular group mating and mating of non-related animals within the frame of the breeding scheme were applied. In 1993 and 2003 average coefficients of inbreeding (F_x) were calculated from 5 parental generations for stallions and mares in the whole breed, white and black variety and sire lines within the varieties. From 1993 to 2003 decreased the F_x (%) for stallions in the: breed from 7.16 to 5.47, white variety from 6.06 to 5.1, black variety from 8.21 to 5.94 and for mares in the: breed from 7.9 to 5.05, white variety from 7.29 to 4.17 and black variety from 8.4 – 5.86. The variation of F_x (%) in the sire lines was for stallions between 2.01 and –7.9 and for mares between 2.21 and –5.72. The majority of sire lines showed a reduction in the F_x.

Keywords: Old Kladrub horse, structure and development, rate of inbreeding, dam fertility, polymorphism

Introduction

The Old Kladrub horse is an important Czech horse breed, which fulfills most of the criteria for genetic resources. The breed existing today is a warmblood created on the basis of Old Spanish and Old Italian horses and bred continuously in the Czech Republic for more than two hundred years. The breed is a robust carriage (coach) horse, which was originally used for ceremonial purposes by the Habsburg emperors. The breeding population is located in the middle of Bohemia and in the southern parts of Moravia. Today the population is divided into 5 gray lines (GENERALE, GENERALISSIMUS, SACRAMOSO, FAVORY, RUDOLFO) and 5 black lines (SACRAMOSO, SOLO, SIGLAVY PAKRA, ROMKE, GENERALISSIMUS). The Old Kladrub horse can be traced back to the founder sires, which represent sire lines existing today (Table 1).

From the very beginning it has been a population of limited number and because of this inbreeding took place over centuries and especially in the past decades. Inbreeding in its conseqequences could lead to inbreeding depression, especially in characters related to fitness (reproduction traits). This is why it is necessary, in the framework of repeated genetic analyses, to pay attention to the rate of inbreeding. Volenec *et al.* (1995) carried out a study of the rate of inbreeding in the Old Kladrub horse. As a result of this analysis the population was closed against gene immigration from related breeds of Old Spanish origin.

Table 1. Survey of founder sires.

No.	Name	Variety	Date of birth	Breed	Origin
1	Generale	Grey	1787	Old Kladrub	Kopčany stud (Moravia)
2	Generalissimus I	Grey	1797	Old Kladrub	Son of Generale (Kopčany)
3	Sacramoso	Black	1800	Old Kladrub	Kroměříž stud (Moravia)
4	Napoleone	Black	1845	Old Kladrub	Rome – line ceased in 1922
5	Solo	Black	1927	Old Kladrub	Son of Sacramoso XXIX
6	Favory	Grey	1938	Lipizzan[1]	Bábolna stud (Hungary)
7	Siglavy Pakra	Black	1946	Lipizzan[1]	Lipica stud (Slovenia)
8	Romke	Black	1966	Friesian[1]	The Netherlands
9	Rudolfo	Grey	1968	Lusitano[1]	Portugal

[1]breeds of Old Spanish origin

The objective of the paper is to analyse the development and the rate of inbreeding of the Old Kladrub breed within the period from 1993 to 2003.

Material and methods

The structure of the breeding animals in the year 2003 (colour varieties, sires and dams) was analysed. Coefficients of inbreeding were calculated for all horses (stallions and mares) from the information of 5 generations of ancestors according to Wright (1922). The genetic analysis was carried out in the year 2003 in the same way as in the year 1993. For the calculation of inbreeding coefficients a special software was developed. The individual coefficients of inbreeding were used for the calculation of average coefficients of inbreeding for various groups of animals (whole population, varieties, sex and lines). The actual results of the analysis (2003) were compared with those obtained in 1993 and the shift in the rate of inbreeding within this 10-year breeding period was analysed.

The coefficients of inbreeding were used as a measure of the dispersive process. The effective population size (N_e), variance of the change of gene frequency ($\sigma^2_{\wedge q}$) and expected increment of inbreeding (ΔF) in one generation were calculated according to Falconer & Mackay (1996). To find out if the Old Kladrub breed is endangered by the inbreeding depression the fertility of dams was analysed in the time span from 1995 to 2003.

The counterpart of the mathematical tools for describing the genetic diversity are genetic methods which analyse the frequencies of alleles. Differences in these frequencies were shown by different types of markers: bloodtypes, biochemical markers, microsatellites, which were published by Jakubec *et al.* (1996) and Hořín *et al.* (1998).

Results and discussion

Development of the breed

The structure of the breeding animals of the Old Kladrub horse in the years 1993 and 2003 (colour varieties, sires and dams) is shown in Table 2 and 3. The breeding population consists of 389 breeding horses (39 sires and 350 dams) in 2003. Within the 10-year breeding period (1993-2003) the number of sires increased from 33 to 39 (Table 2). This increment was only slight, and it was due to the increase of sires in the grey variety (from 16 to 22). The number of sires in the black variety was the same (17) in both years 1993 and 2003. During the same period the number of mares increased from 209 (95 grey and 114 black) to 350 (169 grey and 181 black) – Table 3.

Effective population size

The effective population size, calculated according to Falconer & Mackay (1996) increased from N_e = 114.00 (1993) to N_e = 140.36 (2003). The increment of N_e during the 10 year period was 26.36 animals. From the effective population size we can see that the breed was endangered in both years (1993 and 2003). The generation interval corresponds approximately to 10 years in the Old Kladrub horse. If random mating were applied, the rate of inbreeding with respect to the number of sires and dams would be 0.44 % in 1993 and 0.36 % in 2003.

Rate of inbreeding

Stallions

Table 2 shows average inbreeding coefficients of stallions within both varieties and sire lines in 1993 and 2003. The average coefficient of inbreeding for the whole population and in both varieties of the breeding stallions remained within the 10-year period almost unchanged despite the matings between as far as possible unrelated stallions and mares and realized circular group mating. This phenomenon can be explained by the fact, that when stallions were selected for breeding emphasis was first of all put on the results of the performance test and conformation evaluation. Within this period for all grey sire lines the decrease of F_x from 6.06 % to 5.20 % (-1.06 %) was recorded. The average coefficient of inbreeding increased in the black sire lines from 5.26 % to 5.94 % (0.68 %).

Table 2. Average inbreeding coefficients (F_x) in % of stallions within sire lines and both varieties in 1993 and 2003.

Variety	Sire line	1993		2003		Difference	Min.[1]	Max.[1]
		n	F_x (%)	n	F_x	F_x	F_x	F_x
Grey	Generale	2	11.25	5	7.03	- 4.22	0.00	9.57
	Generalissimus	3	8.23	4	3.86	- 4.37	1.95	5.86
	Favory	6	2.42	6	4.82	2.40	1.56	7.23
	Rudolfo	2	7.25	2	2.64	- 4.61	2.53	2.73
	Sacramoso	3	6.93	5	5.47	-1.46	3.32	7.23
	Average	16	6.06	22	5.20	-1.06	0.00	9.57
Black	Sacramoso	5	1.06	6	9.44	8.38	4.69	11.72
	Solo	6	7.83	7	5.08	- 2.75	2.34	8.98
	Siglavy Pakra	3	4.50	2	3.61	-0.89	2.73	8.98
	Romke	3	7.90	1	0.00	-7.90	0.00	0.00
	Generalissimus	-	-	1	1.56	1.56	1.56	1.56
	Average	17	5.26	17	5.94	0.68	0.00	11.72
Total	Average	33	5.65	39	5.52	-0.13	0.00	11.72

[1]the minimal and maximal F_x refer to values in 2003

Mares

Table 3 shows average inbreeding coefficients of mares within both varieties and sire lines in 1993 and 2003. The average coefficient of inbreeding for the whole population (grey and black lines) of dams decreased from the value 7.75 % to 4.88 % (-2.87 %) within the 10-year period. The coefficients of inbreeding were reduced in all lines. The highest difference was found in the lines RUDOLFO (-5.89 %) and SACRAMOSO (-4.68 %) and the lowest difference in the lines ROMKE (-0.25 %) and FAVORY (-0.84 %). Obviously two main reasons were responsible for this decrease of the coefficient of inbreeding. The first one was the application of circular group mating. The second one was the rapid dam population growth after a bottleneck situation in 1993. Within the period of ten years the number of dams increased from 209 to 350, i.e. an increase of 141 dams (67.5 %). Inbreeding (increase of homozygosity) results in a reduced *fitness* which is the genetic basis of the phenomenon of *inbreeding depression.* To find out if the Old Kladrub breed is endangered by the process of inbreeding the fertility of dams was analysed in the time span from 1995 to 2003.

Table 3. Average inbreeding coefficients (F_x) in % of mares within sire lines and both varieties in 1993 and 2003.

Variety	Sire line	1993			2003			Differene	Min.[1]	Max.[1]
		Sires n	Dams n	F_x	Sires n	Dams n	F_x	F_x	F_x	F_x
Grey	Generale	2	10	8.59	2	21	6.32	-2.27	2.34	10.55
	Generalissimus	3	28	9.84	1	17	5.89	-3.95	2.54	10.74
	Favory	6	30	4.19	3	77	3.48	-0.71	0.39	13.48
	Rudolfo	2	8	7.29	1	15	1.75	-5.54	0.39	5.66
	Sacramoso	3	19	9.96	3	33	4.24	-5.72	0.39	12.11
	Solo	-	-	-	2	3	2.21	2.21	0.00	6.64
	Siglavi Pakra	-	-	-	1	1	0.20	0.20	0.20	0.20
	Romke	-	-	-	1	2	0.00	0.00	0.00	0.00
	Average	16	95	7.29	14	169	3.99	-3.30	0.00	13.48
Black	Sacramoso	5	24	11.31	3	63	7.26	-4.05	2.34	17.58
	Solo	6	48	8.38	2	66	5.45	-2.93	1.37	17.97
	Siglavi Pakra	3	14	9.21	1	14	6.33	-2.88	2.34	15.82
	Romke	3	28	4.48	1	33	4.49	0.01	2.93	10.55
	Generalissimus	-	-	-	1	5	1.29	1.29	1.95	4.10
	Average	17	114	8.40	8	181	5.86	-2.54	1.37	17.97
Total	Average	33	209	7.75	22	350	4.88	-2.87	0.00	17.97

[1]the minimal and maximal F_x refer to values in 2003

Dam fertility

The fertility of dams was analysed separately in the grey and black variety within the National stud at Kladruby and private studs from 1995 and 2003. The results of this analysis for both varieties are shown in Table 4. The fertility rate of both varieties and both types of studs is 65.34 % and the fertility rate values are within the span of 60.23 % in 1996 and 71.84 % in 1997. The lowest fertility rate of 55.91 % was recognized in the private farms in 1996 and the highest fertility rate of 73.33 % was found in the National stud in 1997. The difference between the lowest and highest value was 17.42 %. No tendency caused by the inbreeding depression was found in the fertility rate within the period of 1995 and 2003.

Table 4. Fertility of the grey and black Old Kladrub mares within the National stud at Kladruby and private studs.

Year	National stud			Private studs			Total		
	Number of mated mares	Number of born foals	Fertility rate %	Number of mated mares	Number of born foals	Fertility rate %	Number of mated mares	Number of born foals	Fertility rate %
1995	114	76	66.67	108	69	63.89	222	145	65.32
1996	83	54	65.06	93	52	***55.91***	176	106	***60.23***
1997	105	77	**73.33**	101	71	**70.30**	206	148	**71.84**
1998	101	68	67.33	115	65	56.52	216	133	61.57
1999	104	72	69.23	102	66	64.71	206	138	66.99
2000	83	54	65.06	111	72	64.86	194	126	64.95
2001	105	69	65.71	100	70	70.00	205	139	67.80
2002	117	79	67.52	120	82	68.33	237	161	67.93
2003	83	51	***61.45***	119	71	59.66	202	122	60.40
Average	99.44	66.67	67.05	107.67	68.67	63.78	207.11	135.33	65.34

Polymorphism of bloodtypes, biochemical markers and microsatellites

Jakubec *et al.*, 1996 and HOŘIN *et al.*, 1998 tested stallions and mares of different age for 7 systems of bloodtypes (A, C, D, K, P, Q and U), 5 systems of genetic variants in the serum or plasma - ALB (albumin), TF (transferrin), ES (carboxylesterase), GC (vitamin D binding protein), A1B (β- glycoprotein) and 5 systems in red blood cells - HBA (haemoglobin), GPI (glucose phosphate isomerase), PGD (6-phosphogluconatedehydrogenase), PGM (phosphoglucomutase); CA (carbonic anhydrase) - only Jakubec *et al.* (1996) and Pi (protease inhibitor) – only Hořín *et al.* (1998).

The individuals were in both cases grouped into both colour varieties (grey and black). The average heterozygosity was estimated according to Nei & Roychoudhuri (1974). The result of the analysis is specified in Table 5. Hořín *et al.* (1998) found higher values of the average heterozygosity (0.44) at blood type and biochemical loci than Jakubec *et al.* (1996) (0.34). The average heterozygosity of microsatellites (0.65) was much higher than in the blood type and biochemical loci (0.34 resp. 0.44). The average heterozygosity in the breed was enough large and was connected with a low coefficient of inbreeding.

Table 5. Average heterozygosity at blood type, biochemical and mSat loci in the Kladrub breed (Hořín et al., *1998 and Jakubec* et al., *1996).*

Variety	Hořín *et al.*, 1998					Jakubec *et al.*, 1996	
	n	Blood type loci	Biochemical loci	Average	Microsatellite loci	n	Average (blood type and bio-chemical loci)
Grey	63	0.47	0.34	0.41	0.67	73	0.31
Black	73	0.53	0.42	0.48	0.64	109	0.36
Total	136	0.50	0.38	0.44	0.65	182	0.34

Acknowledgement

The authors gratefully acknowledge the financial support of the project MSM-412100001

References

Falconer, D.S. and T.F.C. Mackay, 1996. Introduction into quantitative genetics. Longman House, Harlow, Essex, 464pp.
Hořín, P., E.G. Cothran, K. Trtková, E. Marti, V. Glasnák, P. Henney, M. Vyskočil, 1998. Polymorphism of Old Kladruber horses, a surviving but endangered baroque breed. Europ. J.Immunogen. 25, 357-363.
Jakubec, V., V. Glasnák, J. Jelínek, J. Přibyl, J. Volenec, N. Záliš, 1996. Genetic analysis of sire lines and sire progeny groups in the Old Kladrub horse. Sci. Agric. Bohem. 27, 283-292.
Volenec, J., V. Jakubec, J. Jelínek, J. Přibyl, N. Záliš, 1995. Analysis of inbreeding of the Old Kladrub horse. Sci. Agric. Bohem. 16, 279-296.
Wright, S., 1922. Coefficients of inbreeding and relationship. Amer. Nat. 56, 330-338.

The numerical and genetic status of native horse and pony breeds in Britain

G.L.H. Alderson

Countrywide Livestock Ltd, 6 Harnage, Shrewsbury SY5 6EJ, United Kingdom

Abstract

Native equine breeds comprise less than 40% of the total horse and pony breeds in Britain. Changing circumstances have diverted equines from agricultural functions to the leisure industry, and have caused stocks of native purebred animals to decline. Support is provided primarily by the Rare Breeds Survival Trust (RBST) and breed societies, assisted by the betting industry. Currently, twelve breeds are listed in RBST categories. Most breeds have experienced introgression at some stage in their development, and some in recent years. The RBST evaluates breeds on the basis of endangerment and between-breed diversity in order to determine prioritisation for allocation of resources in support of native breeds. Research projects have provided valuable data on genetic diversity and breed relationships, which assist the RBST to develop effective strategies for breed conservation.

Keywords: equine breeds, genetic diversity, conservation, rare breeds, distinctive, adaptation

Introduction

The Country Report on Farm Animal Genetic Resources (Defra, 2002), produced within the FAO global 'State of the World Animal Genetic Resources' (SoWAnGR) project, identified 44 equine breeds present in the United Kingdom. Subsequently, a further three breeds were identified, and the final total of 47 breeds comprised 18 (38.3%) native breeds or colour types and 29 (61.7%) exotic breeds. Horses and ponies had been superseded by mechanical power on farms by the mid-20th century, and most breeds have been in serious decline thereafter. They were no longer recognised as part of the agricultural industry, and found new functions in the leisure industry.

The most numerous breed is the Thoroughbred, but the equine industry in the United Kingdom is becoming dominated increasingly by 'sport horses', and this is reflected by a decrease in the numbers of native breeds. Most of these have reached critical levels of endangerment, as evidenced by surveys conducted by the Rare Breeds Survival Trust (RBST) (Table 1). Nine breeds were listed in 2001 (Eriskay, Exmoor, Dales, Dartmoor and Fell ponies, Cleveland Bay, Clydesdale, Shire and Suffolk horses) and subsequently three further breeds (Highland Pony, Welsh Pony A, Hackney Horse) have been added. The Welsh Mountain Pony (Section A) is the foundation for the other three types (Sections B, C and D) of the Welsh Pony and Welsh Cob. It evolved with crosses from the Arab, Thoroughbred and Roadster. The Hackney Horse, with its extravagant action, is descended from the Roadsters (trotting horses) of Yorkshire and Norfolk, based heavily on Thoroughbred foundation animals.

Support for native breeds

Historically, native rare breeds in the United Kingdom have been supported by the RBST and the appropriate breed society. Recently, an increasing volume of legislation and bureaucracy has placed an excessive burden on breed societies, and their authority within the industry has been undermined further by the creation of a National Equine Database (NED). The survival of rare equine breeds currently demands increasing support, and support programmes for native breeds continue to be provided by the RBST. In particular, the 'Horseshoe Appeal' in the 1990s realised circa £100,000 in support of endangered breeds. The Horserace Betting Levy Board (HBLB) also supported non-Thoroughbred breeds from 1970 through grants (Table 1) which served to encourage an increased number of foal registrations.

Prioritisation for support has been determined in different ways. Initially, the HBLB awarded funds in proportion to the size of the animal and the population of the breed (Home Office, 2000). Thus the Shire, a relatively numerous heavy horse, received a significantly higher grant than a more severely threatened small breed such as the Exmoor Pony. The HBLB also awarded grants to two exotic breeds. Subsequently, the HBLB sought to restrict the payment of grants to those breeds recognised by the RBST.

The RBST directed its independent support to native breeds, and gave greatest support to the most endangered breeds. Endangerment is determined primarily by population size, but geographical distribution and genetic structure of the breed are also taken into account. Programmes initiated by the RBST during the 1990s as part of its conservation policy included breed structure analyses, DNA profiling and the creation of a semen archive.

Table 1. HBLB grants to horse and pony breeds in the UK.

Breed	Grant (£) 2001	Mares 2001	RBST status
Eriskay Pony	nil	150	1 critical
Dales Pony	3,220	850	3 vulnerable
Exmoor Pony	3,220	575	2 endangered
Fell Pony	3,300	400	3 vulnerable
Dartmoor Pony	3,520	330	3 vulnerable
Percheron[1]	9,530	n/k	n/a
Irish Draught[1]	9,530	n/k	n/a
Cleveland Bay	10,340	300	1 critical
Suffolk	12,140	69	1 critical
Clydesdale	13,340	500	4 at risk
Shire	35,180	1800	7 minority

[1]Exotic breed

Global populations are taken into account when assessing the degree of endangerment. Most British rare equine breeds are found in small populations elsewhere, but remain globally endangered. On the other hand, some British native breeds, which are not endangered, are recorded as endangered populations in some other countries (Scherf, 2000). The Throughbred is categorised as endangered in Cyprus, Finland, Greece and Yugoslavia, and the Welsh Pony (all Sections) is given the same status in Denmark, Finland and France, but neither breed is endangered either globally or in its country of origin.

Breed relationships

Research has been carried out in the UK, Germany and the USA to determine the place of British breeds in the global equine family. A study of the origins of the domestic horse (Jansen *et al.*, 2002) concluded 'that several distinct horse populations were involved in the domestication of the horse' and that breeds can be grouped in distinct phylogenetic clusters. The study was based on mitochondrial DNA and thus does not show the contribution of exotic stallions to the evolution of local breeds, but the maternal element exhibits strong geographical characteristics. One cluster contains a high proportion of animals derived from Barb (North Africa) and Iberian stock, including American mustangs. Another contains only pony breeds from the British Isles, Scandinavia and central Europe, including Exmoor, Highland, Fjord, Icelandic and Connemara.

Other workers have reached similar conclusions. An American study (Cothran, 1995), using RAPDs, concluded that breeds fall into natural clusters, which broadly approximate to breeds developed in North America, breeds related to the Arab, breeds related to the Andalusian (Iberian), and northern European breeds - including both heavy horses and ponies. The Iberian and Arab groups were most closely related, and the northern European group was the most genetically distant.

A more detailed examination of British breeds does not entirely support these conclusions. Fourteen breeds (including 4 exotic breeds - Irish Draught, Lipizzaner, Akhal Teke and Arab) were included in a study (Crew, 1999) which explored specific relationships between selected breeds in order to advise the RBST's conservation strategy. The breeds fell into four groups - pony breeds, heavy horses, middleweight breeds and 'hot-bloods'. The 'hot-bloods' were related most closely to middleweight breeds, and were most distant from pony breeds, as were the middleweight breeds. This concurs with Cothran's results. The heavy breeds were more closely related to the Arab and middleweight groups than to the pony group, and this does not concur with Cothran's results.

The breeds within the heavy draught group were not closely related, and the Suffolk is related more closely to French and Belgian breeds than to other British heavy breeds. In contrast, other groups were more closely related. The group of middleweight breeds (Cleveland Bay, Irish Draught and Lipizzaner) probably owe their close relationship to their common ancestry through Andalusian and Thoroughbred introgression. The pony breeds, with the exception of the Highland, formed a markedly close-knit group. The Highland showed affinity to both Scottish heavy horses and the Lipizzaner, supporting historical evidence of Clydesdale and Andalusian introgression.

Historically, the RBST has used breed population size (an indicator of endangerment) and genetic distance (an indicator of between-breed diversity) as the two main criteria to determine prioritisation for resources. The measurement of between-breed diversity identifies distinctive breeds and is an important factor in the development of programmes for the conservation of endangered breeds. Numerical data of population - both size and trends - indicate the nature and urgency of support required for each breed. Low within-breed diversity is a feature of many numerically small breeds.

Genetic diversity

Inbreeding, calculated from the recorded pedigree of each individual within a breed, has been used previously as a prime indicator of genetic diversity. The limitations of this measure have diminished its use, and consequently greater attention was given to the correlation between unequal founder effect and the loss of heterozygosity and allelic variability. A proposal to apply effective founder number ($1/\sum P_i^2$) as a measure of genetic conservation (Alderson, 1992) was adopted to demonstrate the influence of the Carthusian strain in the Andalusian breed (Valera, 1997), and subsequently in the analysis of other breeds. Recently, molecular data, such as multi-locus microsatellite genotyping, have played an important role during the last decade in the characterisation of genetic diversity.

Heterozygosity

Genetic erosion occurs more rapidly in small populations as heterozygosity usually is correlated negatively with population size, and many 'rare breeds' show low levels of within-breed diversity. In the British research (Crew, 1999) the level of heterozygosity showed a wide range (Table 2) from 0.47 (Exmoor Pony) and 0.53 (Eriskay Pony) to 0.72 (Irish Draught). The results for these extreme breeds appear to coincide with historical and anecdotal evidence. A study of the breed structure of the Exmoor Pony (Alderson, 1984) showed that one line within the breed (Heatherman 78/2) was becoming dominant, and other studies calculated values for coefficient of inbreeding in moorland (free-living) herds of >35. The Eriskay Pony was derived from a very small founder population in the 1960s, and the breed has a high coefficient of inbreeding. In contrast, the Irish Draught has experienced significant introgression from the Thoroughbred, which has served to increase heterozygosity.

The results for some breeds were unexpected. In particular, the Suffolk showed the second highest level of heterozygosity (0.71), although the entire breed descends from one male line (Crisp's Horse of Ufford 1768) with significant inbreeding. The close breeding has been exaggerated in recent times by a small breeding population, whereby less than 20 foals have been registered each year. The results indicate that a closer scrutiny of breed structure and pedigree data is necessary. However, a high level of breed heterozygosity is not necessarily incompatible with a high level of inbreeding in individual animals, and this probably applies to all the heavy breeds, but especially to the Suffolk.

All the native equine breeds listed by the RBST have suffered a genetic bottleneck in the second half of the twentieth century, and this would be expected to reduce the level of heterozygosity in all cases. For example, the sire lines of the Cleveland Bay of the 1950s and 1960s trace to only one stallion, Wonderful Lad, foaled in 1851 (Walling, 1994), and only 18 Dales Pony foals were registered during a five-year period (1948-1952) (FitzGerald, 2000). Some authors (Cook, 1992) have associated reduced heterozygosity, and related increases in inbreeding in some breeds, with infertility and a high level of genetic defects, such as recurrent laryngeal neuropathy (RLN) in Thoroughbred, Clydesdale and Irish Draught horses, and osteochondrosis dissecans (OCD) in Thoroughbred and Swedish Warmblood horses.

Table 2. Heterozygosity and allelic variability of 14 equine breeds at 10 loci.

Breed	No. samples (n)	Alleles seen (a)	Hetero-zygosity	Alleles 1[1]	Alleles 2[2]
Dales	11	35	0.56	55.53	64.08
Fell	10	33	0.55	53.16	61.73
Eriskay	32	41	0.52	49.43	51.86
Highland	25	43	0.60	56.35	60.64
Exmoor	28	46	0.47	58.12	61.83
Cleveland Bay	30	48	0.65	59.22	62.56
Irish Draught[3]	60	78	0.72	71.24	69.87
Lipizzaner[3]	48	61	0.69	62.17	62.45
Suffolk	70	72	0.71	60.52	58.41
Clydesdale	28	38	0.56	48.01	51.07
Shire	16	39	0.50	57.55	64.53
Akhal Teke[3]	6	32	0.61	54.90	65.57
Arab[3]	50	56	0.63	55.99	56.00
Thoroughbred	74	49	0.61	39.91	38.30

[1]alleles 1 corrected to sample size of 50 animals by $a/(n*0.531+29.457)*56.007$
[2]alleles 2 corrected to sample size of 50 animals by $a/(n*0.7066+25.398)*60.728$
[3]exotic breed

Allelic variability

The variation in the number of animals (samples) tested in each equine breed required a correction factor to be applied to a standard of 50 samples, and the linear correlation between the number of alleles seen and the number of animals tested enabled the calculation of effective corrections for all breeds ('Alleles 1') and all breeds less the Thoroughbred ('Alleles 2') (Table 2). Allelic variability was tested at 10 loci, and the corrected number of alleles seen in the samples for each breed varied from 40 to 71. It is not possible to reconcile these results entirely with the levels of heterozygosity calculated (Crew, 1999) or with historical records of genetic bottlenecks. However, to put them in context, results from some other breeds show even lower allelic variability. White Park cattle (98 samples tested at 11 loci) exhibited an average of 5.1 alleles per locus, compared with an average of 5.6 alleles per locus for 50 samples of each equine breed. The ancient White Park breed, which is descended from 76 founders but owes circa 80% of its ancestry to only eight founders (Alderson, 1997), experienced a severe genetic bottleneck 1940-1975 (N_e circa 22), and has low heterozygosity (0.54). It provides a useful comparison for endangered equine breeds.

The low level of allelic variability in the Thoroughbred demonstrates that small population is not necessarily the main cause of genetic erosion. The intensive single-purpose selection of Thoroughbred horses has caused a significant loss of alleles, which may account partly for the possibility that the breed seems to have reached a genetic plateau. Only ten founder animals (from a total of circa 80 founders) contribute 50% of the ancestry of the breed. This position is mirrored closely by the ubiquitous Holstein in the dairy cattle industry, where the dominance of a cohort of related bulls has similarly reduced genetic variability.

Analysis of endangered native breeds in Britain

Heavy breeds

Suffolk

The genetic distance of the Suffolk from all other breeds, including other British heavy draught breeds, reinforces its status as a distinctive breed. It exhibits a surprising level of heterozygosity and allelic variation in view of its small population size (currently N_e 41.7) over many generations, but it is awarded high priority because of its low numbers and distinctiveness.

Shire and Clydesdale

The physical similarity of these two breeds, and the documented exchange of breeding animals between them, would indicate a close relationship. In 1942 a reciprocal grading-up scheme was agreed to fast-track progeny of crosses with the other breed (Chivers, 1976) and genetic exchange has continued. However, a close relationship is not supported by the measurement of genetic distance (0.577), and they are clearly distinct breeds. The Clydesdale is much closer to the Highland Pony (genetic distance 0.296).

Middleweight breeds

Cleveland Bay

In the early stages of the formation of the Cleveland Bay as a recognisable breed, Iberian (Andalusian) influence was the most notable feature, and this may account for close relationship to the Lipizzaner (genetic distance 0.386). Subsequently Thoroughbred introgression became the dominant factor, as it was in the Irish Draught, and this is confirmed by the close genetic relationship between the Cleveland Bay and the Thoroughbred (genetic distance 0.349). In contrast to the Clydesdale/Highland geographical relationship, the Cleveland Bay and the Dales Pony are genetically distant (0.904) despite their geographical proximity.

Hackney Horse

No genetic data have been accumulated at this stage for the Hackney Horse, but a close relationship to the Thoroughbred is assumed.

Pony breeds

Eriskay and Highland

The Eriskay is a recently discovered breed, with only a very small group of founders, which may represent the former Western Isles type of Highland Pony. The Highland on the mainland is an older breed, but has experienced introgression from several sources, including Spanish, Arab, Roadsters and Clydesdale. The Eriskay is related closely to all the other pony breeds, but the Highland is not related to other pony breeds (except the Eriskay) and is much more closely related to the Clydesdale (genetic distance 0.296), a neighbouring Scottish heavy breed. The Eriskay is recognised by the RBST as a separate breed with high priority. Its small founder population is reflected in a low level of heterozygosity, and low allelic variation.

Dales and Fell

The Dales and Fell are neighbouring pony breeds, which have their area of origin in the Pennine hills, on the eastern slopes and western slopes respectively. There are records of exchange of breeding animals between the breeds in the first half of the twentieth century, and this is evident in their close genetic relationship (genetic distance 0.289). Both breeds owe part of their ancestry to the extinct Galloway, and maybe to the Friesian in post-Roman Britain, but the Fell is a more distinctive breed which has suffered less introgression. It is significantly distant genetically from breeds in all groups, especially the Thoroughbred (1.008), Suffolk (1.096) and Highland (1.034). Significant Clydesdale influence on the Dales Pony has been postulated, but their genetic distance (0.606) does not support this contention.

Exmoor and Dartmoor

Both these breeds maintain free-living moorland herds in their original locality but, while the Exmoor has remained relatively protected from introgression, stallions of other breeds are permitted to run on Dartmoor. The survival of the moorland herds is essential to conserve the native adaptation of the breeds, as other selection pressures direct the development of non-moorland herds. The Exmoor is an ancient British breed, with distinctive features. It is closely related to the Fell but not to the Dales (genetic distances 0.385 and 0.707 respectively) and to the Eriskay but not to the Highland (genetic distances 0.353 and 0.695 respectively), but not to any other native breeds.

Welsh Mountain

No genetic data have been accumulated at this stage for the Welsh Mountain Pony (i.e. Section A) in Britain, but historic introgression from several sources is likely to have rendered it a less typical member of the British pony group. Other data (Cothran, 2004) indicate a relationship of the Welsh Pony (Sections not specified) to Norwegian Fjord, Shetland Pony and Icelandic Horse.

Conclusions

Census data of equine breeds in Britain indicate that most native breeds declined numerically in the second half of the twentieth century, and have been required to adapt to new circumstances and new functions. Recent legislation has introduced extra impositions on breed societies, and is likely to cause further decline. The endangered native breeds are supported by the RBST, but need to discover viable ongoing functions to ensure their wellbeing. Data from research projects enhance the ability of the RBST to develop effective prioritisation and conservation programmes. Based on the criteria of number of breeding animals, genetic distance, heterozygosity and allelic variability, the Fell and Exmoor ponies and Suffolk horse deserve the highest priority, although the Eriskay Pony and Cleveland Bay are also numerically threatened.

References

Alderson, G.L.H., 1984. Exmoor Pony Breed Structure. Report to the Exmoor Pony Society, Dulverton.

Alderson, G.L.H., 1992. A System to Maximise the Maintenance of Genetic Variability in Small Populations. In: Alderson, L. and I. Bodo (editors), Genetic Conservation of Domestic Livestock (volume II). CAB International, Wallingford: 18-29

Alderson, L., 1997. A Breed of Distinction. Countrywide Livestock, Shrewsbury, 167 pp.

Chivers, K., 1976. The Shire Horse. J.A. Allen, London, 834 pp.

Cook, W.R., 1992. Some problems relating to the genetic welfare of the middle weight horse breeds in the British Isles. In: Alderson, L. and I. Bodo (editors), Genetic Conservation of Domestic Livestock (volume II). CAB International, Wallingford: 192-204

Cothran, E.G., 1995. Genetic Markers and Breed Identification in Genetic Conservation. In: Crawford, R.D., E.E. Lister and J.T. Buckley (editors), Conservation of Domestic Animal Genetic Resources. Rare Breeds International, Rome: 291-306

Cothran, E.G., 2004. Genetic analysis of the Lac La Croix Indian Pony. Genesis, 19 No 3, 7-9.
Crew, V.K., 1999. A population genetics study of rare British equine breeds. PhD thesis, University of Reading, 478 pp.
Defra, 2002. UK Country Report on Farm Animal Genetic Resources 2002. Department for Environment Food and Rural Affairs, London. 81 pp.
FitzGerald, I., 2000. Dales Ponies. Whittet Books, Stowmarket, 205 pp.
Home Office, 2000. A Consultation Paper on the Proposed Abolition of the Horserace Betting Levy Board and the Licensing of the Racecourse Betting and Pool Betting on Horseracing. Home Office, London. 13 pp.
Jansen, T., P. Forster, M.A. Levine, H. Oelke, M. Hurles, C. Renfrew, J. Weber and K. Olek, 2002. Mitochondrial DNA and the origins of the domestic horse. Proceedings of the National Academy of Sciences, 99 No 16, 10905-10910.
Scherf, B.D. (editor), 2000. World Watch List (3rd edition). FAO, Rome, 726 pp.
Valera, M., 1997. Mejora Genética del Caballo de P.R.E. de Estripe Cartujana. PhD thesis, University of Cordoba.
Walling, G., 1994. An analysis of the breed structure in the Cleveland Bay horse and a plan for the maximal maintenance of its genome. PhD thesis, University of Liverpool.

Characterisation of several Connemara Pony populations

D. Feely, P. Brophy and K. Quinn

University College Dublin, Department of Animal Science and Production, Faculty of Agriculture, Belfield, Dublin 4, Ireland

Abstract

The Connemara Pony is one of Irelands few indigenous equine breeds. It is a numerically small breed, with approximately 2,000 breeding females and 250 breeding males in Ireland. The Department of Agriculture and Food in Ireland have classified the breed as endangered.

The results generated from a characterisation of the population in Ireland indicate that past breeding practices have caused a substantial loss in the breeds' genetic diversity. As a consequence of that project a study was undertaken to characterise and compare the genetic diversity of Connemara Pony populations outside Ireland. Included in this study were the Connemara Pony populations of the United Kingdom, France, North America, Sweden, Denmark and Finland respectively.

Results indicated that, to varying degrees, the level of genetic diversity in the different populations has been in a state of decline. The average inbreeding and relationship coefficient for each reference population ranges from 4.04% and 8.57% in North America, to 4.97% and 19.64% in Finland.

Of the six countries under study North America was the furthest removed from the Irish Connemara Pony population, with the sires of the North American reference population having the lowest average relationship to the sires (6.64%) and dams (6.64%) of the Irish population. Thus, of all of the countries under study the North America Connemara Pony population represents the most likely source of genetic variation, which could be used to widen the gene pool of the Connemara Pony population in Ireland.

Introduction

The Connemara Pony is numerically a small breed, with approximately 2,000 breeding females and 250 breeding males in Ireland. Traditionally, the Connemara was a working pony and enjoyed a prominent role in agricultural life in the West of Ireland. However, in the middle of the last century farming practices changed, and as machinery was introduced, the role of the working pony became redundant. The Connemara Pony has maintained its popularity by establishing a position in the showing and riding industry.

The Connemara Pony Breeders' Society was founded in 1923. Since its formation, the society has been responsible for the maintenance and publication of the Connemara Pony Stud Book. An export market to the United Kingdom and United States developed for the breed in the 1940's and by the 1960's Connemara Ponies were being exported all over Europe. Currently there are 16 different countries, outside Ireland, that have formed their own Connemara Pony Breeders' Societies.

The Irish Connemara Pony Stud Book has been closed since 1964 and the practice of overusing popular sires is prevalent throughout the history of the breed. In 2003 a characterisation of the Connemara Pony population in Ireland was carried out in order to establish how past breeding practices have affected the genetic composition of the current pony population (Feely, 2003). The results generated from the study indicated that past breeding practices had caused a substantial loss in the Irish population's genetic diversity. As the gene pool in the Irish population is relatively narrow it was considered important to analyse the genetic composition of Connemara Pony populations outside Ireland.

The aim of this study was to characterise the Connemara Pony populations of the United Kingdom, France, North America, Sweden, Denmark and Finland. Specific emphasis was placed on how these populations differed from the Irish population. The relationship between the sires in the various countries and the Irish population was calculated in an attempt to identify possible sources of genetic variability that could be used to widen the gene pool of the Irish population.

Materials and methods

Data description

Data from all registered Connemara Ponies from the various countries under study were analysed. A reference population for each country was defined as all purebred foals born between 1998 and 2001 inclusive. The number of animals in each dataset and the reference population is shown in Table 1.

Table 1. The number of records in the dataset and reference population for each country.

Country	No of records in dataset	No of records in reference population
Ireland	20,032	2,844
United Kingdom	5,368	611
North America	3,288	349
France	11,304	2,240
Sweden	4,552	431
Denmark	2,547	209
Finland	424	54

Statistical methods

Data cleaning, inbreeding and relationship coefficients were calculated using SAS® software (SAS® Language and Procedures, 1989). Parameters derived from the probabilities of gene origin and pedigree completeness levels were estimated using the software *Pedig*, which was developed for the pedigree analysis of large populations (Boichard, 2002).

Results

Pedigree completeness

As the accuracy of the genetic characterisation is dependant on the quality of the pedigree information it was imperative that pedigrees were traced back to their earliest known ancestor. The complete generation equivalent (CGE) was used as a measure the level of pedigree completeness for each country giving the average number of complete generations recorded for the animals in the reference populations.
The level of pedigree completeness was very similar across all countries ranging from 6.36 in the UK, to 6.97 in Denmark (see Table 2).

Table 2. The complete generation equivalent, average inbreeding coefficient and average relationship coefficient for the animals in the reference populations.

Country	CGE	Ave inbreeding coefficient	Ave relationship coefficient
Ireland	6.59	4.65%	10.66%
UK	6.36	4.44%	9.29%
N. America	6.38	4.04%	8.57%
France	6.48	4.17%	8.91%
Sweden	6.66	4.72%	11.53%
Denmark	6.97	4.18%	12.84%
Finland	6.75	4.97%	19.64%

Inbreeding

The level of inbreeding in a population is measured by the inbreeding coefficient (Falconer, 1989). The coefficient of inbreeding measures the probability that an animal receives identical genes by descent from its sire and dam.

Finland had the highest level of inbreeding at 4.97%. This was higher than the level of inbreeding detected in the Irish population (4.65%). North America had the lowest level of inbreeding at 4.04%. The level of inbreeding for each country is illustrated in Table 3.

Table 3. The number of founders (f), effective number of founders (f_e), effective number of ancestors (f_a) and the (f_e)/(f_a) ratio for the individuals in the reference populations.

Country	No founders (f)	Effective no of founders (f_e)	Effective no of ancestors (f_a)	Ratio (f_e)/(f_a)
Ireland	351	35.8	18	1.99
UK	353	36.5	18.9	1.93
N.America	331	37.7	23.6	1.6
France	346	40	20.25	1.98
Sweden	184	37.4	18.2	2.05
Denmark	137	41.9	18.08	2.31
Finland	127	35.2	8.35	4.22

Average relationship coefficient

The average relationship coefficient measures the proportion of genes that animals have in common (Crow, 1986).

Finland had the highest relationship among individuals in the reference population, at 19.64%. This high average relationship is due to the large number of half siblings in the reference population. Denmark and Sweden also had high relationship coefficients among the foals in their reference populations. North America has the lowest relationship among the individuals in the reference population (8.57%). Relationship coefficients for each country are given in Table III.

Probabilities of gene

The total number of founders (f), effective number of founders (f_e) and effective number of ancestors (f_a) were estimated using the methods described in Boichard *et al.*, (1997), and are illustrated on Table 3.

For each population the effective number of founders was considerably lower than the actual number of founders. This discrepancy between the actual number of founders and the effective number of founders is expected to decrease the level of genetic diversity in the current populations relative to what would have transpired had all founders contributed equally.

A large $(f_e)/(f_a)$ ratio is indicative of a narrow bottleneck in the population. Bottlenecks occur when a population experiences a period in time when the number of breeding animals is considerably reduced. Finland had the highest $(f_e)/(f_a)$ ratio illustrating a considerable bottleneck in the population. North America has the lowest $(f_e)/(f_a)$ ratio, implying that the North American population's genetic diversity was least effected by past bottlenecks in the population.

Relationship to the Irish population

The average relationship coefficient between the sires of the reference populations of the UK, France, North America, Sweden, Denmark and Finland and the sires and dams of the Irish reference population were estimated in an attempt to identify the countries whose sires are the least related to the breeding population in Ireland (Table 4.). The stallions with the lowest relationship to the dams of the Irish reference population were also identified.

Table 4. The relationship coefficient between the sires of all the reference populations and the Irish sires and dams, and the relationship coefficient of the sire, from each country, that was least related to the Irish dams.

Sires	Irish Sires	Irish Dams	Minimum relationship to Irish dams
Ireland	10.64%	10.15%	5.41%
UK	8.62%	9.03%	4.18%
N.America	6.64%	6.64%	1.09%
France	8.36%	8.2%	4.99%
Sweden	8.4%	8.51%	5.88%
Denmark	7.981%	8.03%	5.57%
Finland	7.663%	7.89%	5.18%

The sires of the North American reference population were the least related to the stallions and dams that produced the Irish reference population.

The stallion with the lowest relationship to the Irish dams was *Gilnocky Drumcliffe*. This stallion, who was bred in the United States, had an average relationship of 1.09% with the dams of the Irish population.

Conclusion

Following the characterisation of the Connemara Pony populations of the United Kingdom, France, North America, Sweden, Denmark and Finland, it is apparent that, to varying degrees, the level of genetic diversity in the different populations has been in a state of decline. In some countries a limited population size has proven detrimental, and in others unbalanced founder and ancestor contributions have been responsible for a reduction in genetic diversity.

The Connemara Pony population in Finland is very small, with approximately 20 foals produced per year. Of the six countries under study Finland had the highest level of inbreeding and relationship among the individuals in the reference population. Given that the future breeding population is very closely related to each other it is vitally important that the genetic diversity of the Connemara Pony population in Finland is carefully managed in future generations. Without the implementation of a well-managed breeding strategy a substantial rise in the level of inbreeding is likely.

North America had the lowest level of inbreeding of the countries under study at 4.04%. The relationship among the animals in the reference population was also lowest in the North American population.

Of the six countries under study North America was the furthest removed from the Irish Connemara Pony population. The sires of the North American dataset had the lowest average relationship to the sires and dams of the Irish population. The stallion that was the least related to the dams of the Irish population, *Gilnocky Drumcliffe,* was included in the North American dataset. Thus, of all of the countries under study the North America Connemara Pony population represents the most likely source of genetic variation, which could be used to widen the gene pool of the Connemara Pony population in Ireland.

Although *Gilnocky Drumcliffe* had the lowest average relationship to the dams of the Irish population there were also stallions in Ireland that had a low relationship to the dams of the Irish reference population. The Irish stallion *Ard Harlequin* had an average relationship coefficient of 5.41% with the dams of the Irish reference population. This suggests that although there are Connemara Pony stallions outside Ireland that harbour a source of genetic variation, there are individual stallions in Ireland that also represent an important source of genetic diversity which could help widen the gene pool of the Irish Connemara Pony population.

Acknowledgements

We would like to thank the Department of Agriculture and Food who funded this project under the Advisory Committee of the Conservation of Genetic Resources for Food and Agriculture. The authors wish to thank the Connemara Pony Breeders' Societies from all of the countries involved in the project for their assistance and for supplying the records used in the analysis.

References

Boichard, D., 2002. Pedig: A FORTRAN Package for pedigree analysis suited for large populations. Proceedings of the 7th World Congr. Genet. Appl. Livest. Prod. CD-ROM Communication n° 28-13.

Boichard, D., L. Maignel and É. Verrier, 1997. The value of using probabilities of gene origin to measure genetic variability in a population. Genetics Selection Evolution 29: 5-23.

Crow, J.F., 1986. Basic Concepts in Population, Quantitative, and Evolutionary Genetics. W. H. Freeman and Company.

Falconer, D.S., 1989. Introduction to quantitative genetics. Longman Scientific and Technical.

Feely, D., 2003. Characterisation of the Connemara Pony population in Ireland. Masters thesis. University College Dublin.

SAS Institute Inc., 1989. SAS® Language and Procedures: Usage, Version 6, First Edition. Cary, NC: SAS Institute Inc., 1989.

Genetic characterisation of the Croatian autochthonous horse breeds based on polymorphic blood proteins and mtDNA data

A. Ivanković[1], P. Dovč[2], P. Caput[1], P. Mijić[3] and M. Konjačić[1]

[1]*Dep. of Animal Production, Faculty of Agriculture, Svetošimunska 25, 10000 Zagreb, Croatia*
[2]*Department of Animal Science, Biotechnical Faculty, Groblje 3, 1230 Domžale, Slovenia*
[3]*Dep. for Zootechnics, Faculty of Agriculture, Trg Sv. Trojstva 3, 31000 Osijek, Croatia*

Abstract

Coldblood horse breeds in Croatia, differentiated in three breeds (Croatian Coldblood, Murinsulaner and Posavina horse), belong to the group of autochthonous endangered breeds. Genetic polymorphisms at the protein- and DNA-level can be successfully used for population analysis and for establishing relationships within and among breeds (populations). Mitochondrial DNA has been frequently used as a marker system in population and evolutionary studies. In this study, by analysing polymorphic blood proteins and mitochondrial DNA, we investigated the genetic structure of the coldblooded horses in Croatia, made an attempt to determine genetic distance between populations and within other cognition horse breeds. Our results show relatively high genotypic diversity within and between three autochthonous horse breeds in Croatia. Our molecular data nicely support phenotypic differentiation between Posavina horse on one side and Croatian Coldblood and Murinsulaner horse on the other side. These results are the first indicators for genetic profile of mentioned breeds and will stimulate further research and application of molecular data for selection.

Keywords: coldblood horses, autochthonous breeds, genetic structure, diversity

Introduction

Croatian coldblood horse breeds make the most numerous breed group of horses in Croatia (approximately 70% of the total horse population). This group of horses has been differentiated in three autochthonous breeds: Croatian Coldblood (45%), Posavina horse (54%) and Murinsulaner horse (1%). Their systematic breeding started in the 19th century in Međimurje and then it spread to Podravina, Posavina and parts of Slavonia. They were bred on the then horse population "busak" which, depending on the climate, was differently conformational and genetically profiled. With the aim of improving the conformation of the then "busak", during the 20th century, quality stallions of heavy European horse breeds were imported, primarily of the Noric (the Noriker) , the Percheron and Belgian blood, which were used for "improving" the existing population. The coldblood horse breeds consolidation started fifteen years ago since breeds were badly structured and intercrossed (Ivanković & Caput, 2004). The population of Posavina horse includes a significant small variability of conformation features, mostly conditioned by breeding area. In the Croatian Coldblood population two breed types have been noticed, which as such should be separately observed and supported in breeding. In the first type, the trace of a hundred-year improvement of the original population with the European breeds of heavy horses has been noticed and it has a bigger body frame, rougher head and stronger bone base. The second type of the Croatian Coldblood is a bit lighter, of a smaller head and smaller body frame. The Murinsulaner horse is in the stage of a breeding consolidation, and its limiting factor is a small effective population size.

The Posavina horse and the Croatian Coldblood remained in the marginal pasture areas in a small number which demands a constant monitoring. Murinsulaner horse population is reduced to forty heads which are carefully monitored, while its revitalisation is questionable. It requires the international cooperation of countries in the area of the river Mura.

Determined blood protein allele frequencies are the first indicators of genetic type profiles, which, together with studied exterior properties, help in more precise defining of autochthonous horse breeds. The control region of the mitochondrial DNA (mtDNA) is, due to the high mutation rate, lack of recombinations and maternal inheritance, a very useful marker system in the population- and evolutionary biology. The objectives of this study were to investigate the genetic structure of the Croatian autochthonous horse breeds and establishing the genetic relationships within and among autochthonous horse breeds.

Materials and methods

The research has been 140 horses included (68 Posavina horses, 56 Croatian Coldblood and 16 Murinsulaner horses). Data on polymorphic protein variants and sequences of D-loop region of mtDNA were used for calculating genetic relationships within and among breeds. Blood protein variants were determined by electrophoresis on "cellogel" strips and PAA gels in a discontinuous buffer system. The 5'-end of the mtDNA control region between the $tRNA^{Pro}$ gene and central conserved sequence block was PCR amplified using primers P28 (5'-AGTCTCACCATCAACCCCCAAAGC-3') and HF (5'-CCTGAAGTAGGAACCAGATG-3'). PCR fragments were sequenced using ABI PRISM BigDye Terminator Cycle Sequencing Ready Reaction Kit and ABI PRISMTM 310 Genetic Analyzer (PE Applied Biosystems, MA). Statistical package Arlequin software (Schneider *et al.* 2000) and MEGA (Kumar *et al.*, 2001) were used in data processing.

Results and discusion

The results indicated two allele variants for Hb and Al, and six allele variations for Tf. The allele frequencies are presented in Figure 1.

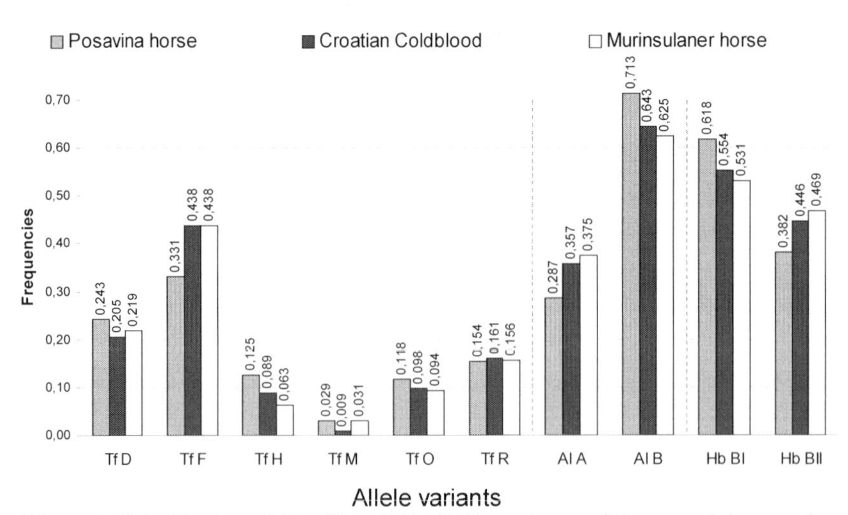

Figure 1. Distribution of Hb, Tf and Al allelic variants of the autochthonous horse breeds in Croatia

The greatest level of heterozygosity was established for Tf (0.6786) and the least for Al (0.5357). The lowest level of heterozygosity was established for the Posavina horse (0.6078), and the greatest for the Murinsulaner horse (0.6667). Measures of genetic variation for each locus are given in Table 1.

Table 1. Number of alleles (No), effective number of alleles (ENA), observed hererozygosity (Ho), expected heterozygosity (He), Shannon's Information index (I), polymorphic informative content (PIC) and average exclusion probability (AEP) polymorphic blood proteins of the autochthonous horse breeds in Croatia.

Locus	No	ENA	Ho	He	I	PIC	AEP
Croatian Coldblood							
Hb	2	1,9773	0,6429	0,4987	0,6874	0,372	0,186
Tf	6	3,6087	0,6250	0,7294	1,4663	0,685	0,501
Al	2	1,8491	0,5714	0,4633	0,6518	0,354	0,177
Average	3,33	2,4784	0,6131	0,5638	0,9352	0,470	$\sum$ 0,666
Posavina horse							
Hb	2	1,8951	0,6176	0,4758	0,6652	0,361	0,180
Tf	6	4,4937	0,7206	0,7832	1,6135	0,744	0,570
Al	2	1,6922	0,4853	0,4121	0,5992	0,325	0,163
Average	3,33	2,6937	0,6078	0,5570	0,9593	0,477	$\sum$ 0,705
Murinsulaner horse							
Hb	2	1,9922	0,6875	0,5241	0,6912	0,374	0,187
Tf	6	3,6056	0,6875	0,7460	1,4877	0,685	0,502
Al	2	1,8824	0,6250	0,4839	0,6616	0,359	0,179
Average	3,33	2,4934	0,6667	0,5813	0,9468	0,473	$\sum$ 0,668

The Posavina horse is phylogenetically more distant from the Murinsulaner horse (0.0176) than from the Croatian Coldblood (0.0124). The genetic distance between the Croatian Coldblood and the Murinsulaner horse is significantly smaller (0.0012), or rather showed a much higher genetic sameness (0.9988).

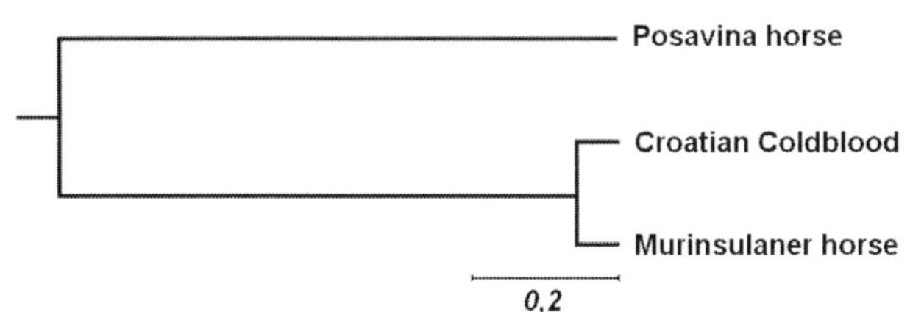

Figure 2. UPGMA Neighbour-Joining tree constructed on the basis of blood protein polymorphism of autochthonous horse breeds in Croatia.

To date, the genetic distances established have not provided a reliable support for the claim of genetic originality of the existing autochthonous horse breeds, but instead suggests a substantial mutual introduction of genomes. The results of typing these genotypes could significantly aid in breeding consolidation, adapting breeding programs and preserving the breed fitness.

Due to its specificity, mitochondrial DNA is an effective marker system in population and evolutionary research (Ishida *et al.* 1995). The structure of D-loop region sequences was investigated in three autochthonous Croatian horse breeds (approximate 353 bp fragment) which are considered to have maintained their autochthonous character.

```
Belgian Coldblood      CCTCATGTGCTATGTCAGTATCAGATTATACCCCCATATAACACCATACCCACCTGACATGCAATATCTTATGAATGGCCTATGTACGTCGTG
Croatian Coldblood     ............................C.......C.....G............................................A.....
Murinsulaner Horse     ....................................C................................................T.A.....
Posavina Horse         ....................................C..................................................A.....
Arabian Horse          ....................................C..................................................A.....
English Thoroughbred   ....................................C...G.............................................TA.....
Belgian Coldblood      CATTAAATTGTTCGCCCCATGAATAATAAGCATGTACATAATATCATTTATCTTACATGAGTACATTATATTATTGATCGTGCATACCCCATC
Croatian Coldblood     ............T................................................................................
Murinsulaner Horse     ...........C.A...............................................................................
Posavina Horse         ............TA...............................................................................
Arabian Horse          ...........CT.............................................AG...............A.................
English Thoroughbred   ............T.............................................AG.................................
Belgian Coldblood      CAAGTCAAATCATTTCCAGTCAACACGCATTATCACAACCCATGTTCCACGAGCTTAATCACCAAGCCGCGGGAAAT
Croatian Coldblood     ..................C..........-....T..........................................
Murinsulaner Horse     .............................-...............................................
Posavina Horse         ..................C..........-..........................G....................
Arabian Horse          .............................-...............................................
English Thoroughbred   ........................T....-...............................................
```

Figure 3. Polymorphic sites within the horse mtDNA D-loop sequence (nt 15498 - 15759; Acc. AF064632, AF132591, AF072990)

These results suggest on the insignificant breed differentiation at the mtDNA level, and indicate significant breed similarities. The mean 'net' distance indicates a greater distance between the Posavina and Murinsulaner horses (0.00198) than between Croatian Coldblood and Posavina horse (-0.00042) and Croatian Coldblood and Murinsulaner horse (-0.00025).

The sequence data from this study were compared with five published sequences of the 261 bp fragment of the mt DNA D-loop region (nt 15498 - 15759) available in the GenBank (*Equs przewalskii* - AccNo. AF014409; English Thoroughbred - AccNo. AF072990; Arabian Horse - AccNo. AF132591; Belgian Coldblood - AccNo. AF064632; Lipizzaner - AccNo. AF168690) in order to demonstrate relationships between some horse breeds (Figure 4).

Table 2. Number of nucleotide differences (lower part) and Jukes-Cantor distances (upper part) among eight sequences of mtDNA (nt 15498 - 15759) found in the subgenus Equus

	Belgian	Cro. Cold.	Murins.	Posav.	Arabian	Thorough.	Lipizz.	*E. Przew.*
Belgian Coldblood	-	0.0312	0.0233	0.0272	0.0312	0.0352	0.0272	0.0272
Croatian Coldblood	8	-	0.0312	0.0193	0.0312	0.0352	0.0312	0.0392
Murinsulaner Horse	6	8	-	0.0193	0.0233	0.0352	0.0233	0.0392
Posavina Horse	7	5	5	-	0.0272	0.0312	0.0272	0.0352
Arabian Horse	8	8	6	7	-	0.0193	0.0000	0.0154
English Thoroughbred	9	9	9	8	5	-	0.0192	0.0272
Lipizzaner	7	8	6	7	0	5	-	0.0154
Equs przewalskii	8	10	10	9	4	7	4	-

Based on these sequence comparisons, a tree presented in Figure 4 was constructed.

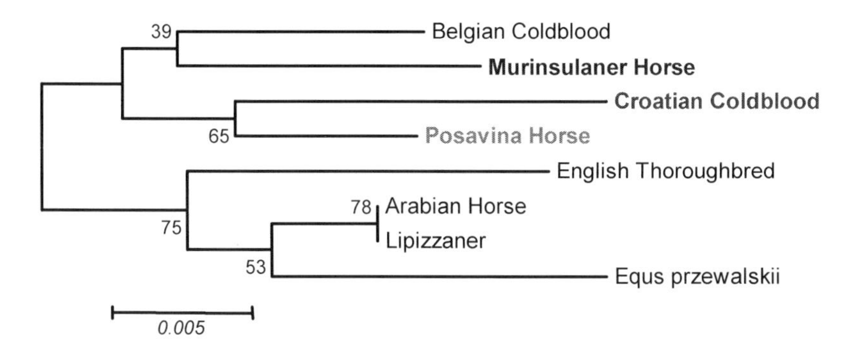

Figure 4. Neighbor-Joining tree of mtDNA D-loop sequences from the members of the genus Equus (Equs przewalskii - AccNo. AF014409; English Thoroughbred - AccNo. AF072990; Arabian Horse - AccNo. AF132591; Belgian Coldblood - AccNo. AF064632; Lipizzaner - AccNo. AF168690)

These observations have to be taken with some restrictions, since the number of researched sequences has been relatively small. The preliminary research mtDNA we need complete the analysis of preponderance of samples along the breed. The completion of existing information by including a higher number of microsatellite loci in studies will give more reliable picture of the phylogenetic relations of observed populations.

Genetic distances alone are sometimes considered as insufficient argument for conservation of the population (Ruane, 1999), but in our case molecular data nicely support genotypic differentiation among populations. Determination of the genetic structure and originality help to determine the most effective model of protection for autochthonous breeds.

Conclusion

Our results show relatively modest genotypic diversity within and between three autochthonous horse breeds in Croatia. Frequencies of polymorphic proteins suggest the larger phylogenetic closeness of the Croatian Coldblood and Muinsulaner horse compared to the Posavina horse. Investigate sequences of the mtDNA suggest of the larger closeness of Posavina horse and Croatian Coldblood, as well as Muinsulaner and Belgian Coldblood horse. Diversity to the sequence mtDNA indicates the significant variability of autochthonous horse breeds in Croatia. These results are the first indicators for genetic profile of mentioned breeds and will stimulate further research and application of molecular data for selection.

Acknowledgement

This study was performed with financial support of the Ministry of Science, Education and Sport of the Republic of Croatia (Project No. 0178-026)

References

GenBank - Database, 2000. NCBI. http://www.ncbi.nlm.nih.gov/

Ishida, N., T. Oyunsuren, S. Mashima, H. Mukoyama and N. Saitou, 1995. Mitochondrial DNA sequences of various species of the genus *Equus* with special reference to the phylogenetic relationship between Przewalskii's Wild Horse and domestic horse. Journal of Molecular Evolution 41, 180-188.

Ivanković, A. and P. Caput, 2004. Exterior features of Croatian autochtonous horse breeds. Stočarstvo 58, 15-36.

Kumar, S., K. Tamura, I.B. Jacobsen and M. Nei, 2001. Molecular Evolutionary Genetics Analysis, Version 2.1.

Ruane, J. 1999. A critical review of the value of genetic distance studies in conservation of animal genetic resources. J. Anim. Breed. Genet. 116, 317-323.

Schneider, S., D. Roessli and L. Excoffier, 2000. Arlequin. Ver 2.000. Genetics and Biometry Lab, Dept. of Anthropology, University of Geneva.

Estimation of genetic distance between traditional horse breeds in Hungary

S. Mihók[1], B. Bán[2], Cs. Józsa[3], and I. Bodó[1]

[1]University of Debrecen Faculty of Agronomy Department of Animal Breeding and Nutrition H-4032 Debrecen Böszörményi út 138
[2]National Institute for Agricultural Quality Control H-1024 Budapest, Keleti Károly-u. 24.
[3]University of Veszprém, Georgikon Faculty of Agricultural Sciences, Department of Physiology and Nutrition, H-8360 Keszthely Deák Ferenc-u 16

Abstract

Modern immuno– and molecular genetic methods are more and more adapted for preservation of traditional animal breeds, horses included. Comparison of blood groups, polymorphic systems and DNA structure of Nonius, Gidran and English Thoroughbred was carried out. These original Hungarian breeds were established at the Mezőhegyes stud more than two centuries ago. Samples of Gidran and Nonius horses were compared to those of Thoroughbred horses. The allele frequency of Gidran breed has shown it to be more homogeneous than the Nonius. The frequency of observed alleles in Gidran and Thoroughbred were more similar compared to Nonius. It corresponds well to the history of the breeds. In some cases the common origin of these two breeds was expressed in the similar alelle frequencies. Furioso-North Star, the Mezőhegyes Halfbred breed will be involved later in the project. Statistical analysis of molecular genetic results helps to estimate gene drift of endangered rare populations. Based upon these results proposals can be elaborated for breeding and mating technics in order to avoid close inbreeding and genetic loss. Estimation of genetic distance between breeds, lines and families is important for breeding strategies and long term decisions.

Introduction

Mezőhegyes in South of Hungary, near to the Maros river, is famous for a big state farm and a former military stud, which should be considered the cradle of three horse breeds born there.

The military stud was established in December 1784, when emperor Josef II accepted the idea of a huge state investment for an estate in order to breed horses for the army. Horses were acquired from Hungary, Transsylvania, Poland Turkey, Moldavia, Caucasus and from Western countries (Hannover, Tschehland, Spain etc). Horses were mainly Spanish or Arabian type animals or good horses from the local population. The most important breeding goal was the utilization in the army, transport and agriculture.

The concept of breed was not developed that time, so the records of the founder horses in the old stud books declare the place of origin and not the breed. The fashion at the end of eighteenth century was the Spanish horse, so most of the horses imported anywhere were Spanish or Neopolitan type.

4-5000 horses were gathered for start. Sanitary problems showed up with the many new acquisitions, therefore from 1814 the farm reduced its population only to the breeding stock. The parentage of foals was recorded with great care, the animals were brand marked and the breeders of present time can admire the precision and correctness of the old handwritten stud books. During the first decads of ninteenth century, the well known Mezőhegyes horse breeds were more and more established because of intensive selection.

Nonius

During the Napoleon wars the Austrian army looted several young stallions from the Rosières stud farm in France. One of them was Nonius, which was sent to Mezőhegyes in 1816. Nonius was an Anglonorman stallion and he was mated to Spanish type mares and this genetic combination proved to be successful. During the period of 1815 - 1832 he covered 368 mares. 79 stallions (15 within the Nonius line) and 122 brood mares were introduced in breeding of the stud. Three generations were enough to fix the characteristics of the Nonius breed : bay, dark bay, or black in colour, roman nose, expressive eyes, steep shoulders, the narrow and short croup, firm skeleton and bones, excellent temperament. Well adaptability for work pretty gait and trot are associated. In order to improve the coarse form of the breed and to balance the effect of inbreeding English Thoroughbred stallions were used later. Four lines were established and combined by intercrossing.

The two World Wars caused a great loss in the animal stock, however, the repair succeeded rapidly. After World War II the horse lost its importance as a military object and later its importance decreased as draught animals as well. In the present situation, the Nonius breed is maintained as a valuable genetic resource for the far future. The number of brood mares in the stud was dramatically reduced and another Nonius stud was established at Hortobágy.

Gidran

The founder of Gidran breed, Gidran senior, a chestnut Arabian stallion was imported from Egypt in 1816 and his son Gidran II bred to several Mezőhegyes mares produced very good progeny. At that time the mares were grouped in different studs according to their coat colour. It appeared, that in the chestnut stud, No. V. the most of the good horses were the descendance of Gidran stallions. It was the reason for establishing a new breed from Gidran progeny. In order to improve their performance Arabian and English Thoroughbred Stallions were used from the second part of ninteenth century and the Gidran became a good breed adaptable also for modern sports, first of all, in eventing.

The Mezőhegyes Halfbred

In the year of 1841, Furioso, an English Thoroughbred stallion born in Hungary, arrived in Mezőhegyes and in 1852 The North Star imported from England started to do his service at the stud. Those two stallions sired many good foals for the bay stud and their male progeny were used as stallions combined in the same populations. The two genealogical lines stabilized the breed, the Mezőhegyes Halfbred (synonym Furioso-North Star) by intercrossing. It is an elegant, noble breed, with voluminous body and good movement. After the losses of two World Wars the regeneration of this breed run with many difficulties, nowadays it can be considered as a good multipurpose horse breed protected in a preservation programme.

Immuno–, and molecular genetic comparison

Modern methods immuno- and molecular genetics are adapted for preservation of traditional domestic animal breeds, horses included. Comparison of blood groups, polymorphic systems and DNA structure of Nonius, Gidran and English Thoroughbred was carried out. The Furioso will be involved later. The comparison of these breeds affords interesting results, because the female basis of the breeds in question was nearly the same or very similar, and the English Thoroughbred as an improver had its role in all the Mezőhegyes breeds, however, more in Gidran and Furioso and not so much in Nonius.

Statistical analysis of molecular genetic results helps to estimate gene drift of endangered rare populations. Based upon these results proposals can be elaborated for breeding and mating technics in order to avoid close inbreeding and genetic loss.

At the blood group investigation only the "D" system was taken into consideration and the following sera were available : Da, b, c, d, e, f, g, h, i, k, l, m, n, o, r. The factors of transferrin, albumin, carboxylesterase, vitamin D binding protein (GC), and A1B glycoprotein (Xk) factors were used.

The collected samples were subjected to PCR and microsatellite analysis. Twelve microsatellites recommended for the parentage control of horses by the International Society for Animal Genetics (ISAG) were determined. Genomic DNA was isolated from lymphocytes by the method described by Marklund *et al* (1994).

The examinations were carried out in the Laboratory of Immunogenetics and DNA of the National Institute for Agricultural Quality Control.

Samples of 55 Gidran, 48 Nonius stallions and mares were compared to those of English Thoroughbred and Standardbred horses. The microsatellite structure of Nonius and Gidran is demonstrated at Figure 1 and 2.

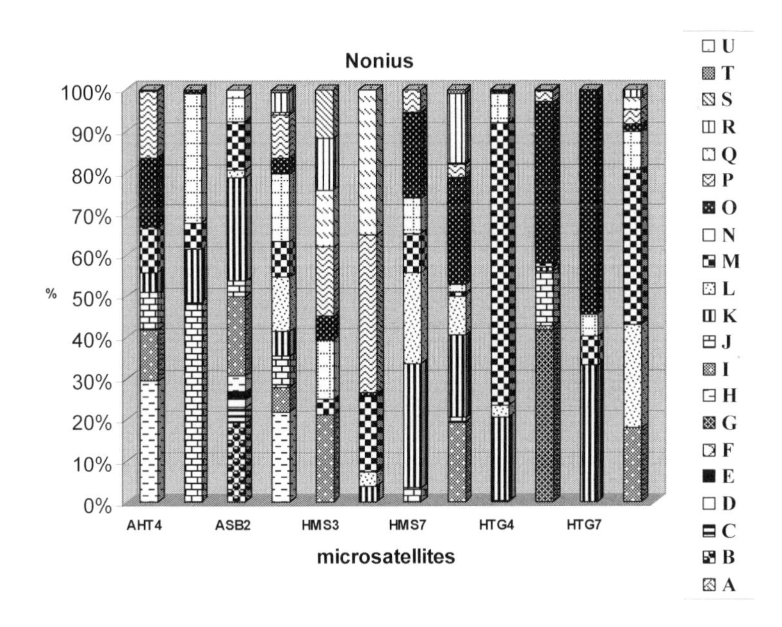

Figure 1. Microsatellite frequencies in Nonius breed.

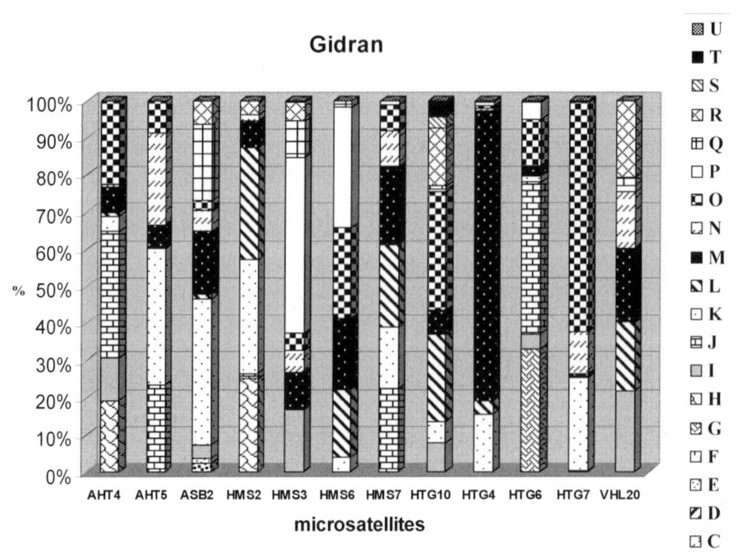

Figure 2. Microsatellite frequencies in Gidran breed.

„D" blood group

In Nonius 11 and in Gidran 9 alleles were observed. In the Nonius *„bcm"* (0,3893) and *„dkl"* (0,175), and in the Gidran *„dkl"* (0,6395) alleles were dominant. The *„cgmr"*, *„dghmr"* and *„dlr"* alleles could not be found in Gidran, which occurs with low frequency in the Nonius breed. The *„adl"* allele was not detectable in Nonius. Both breeds were characterised by the high level of allele frequency.

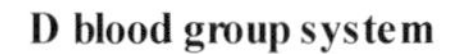

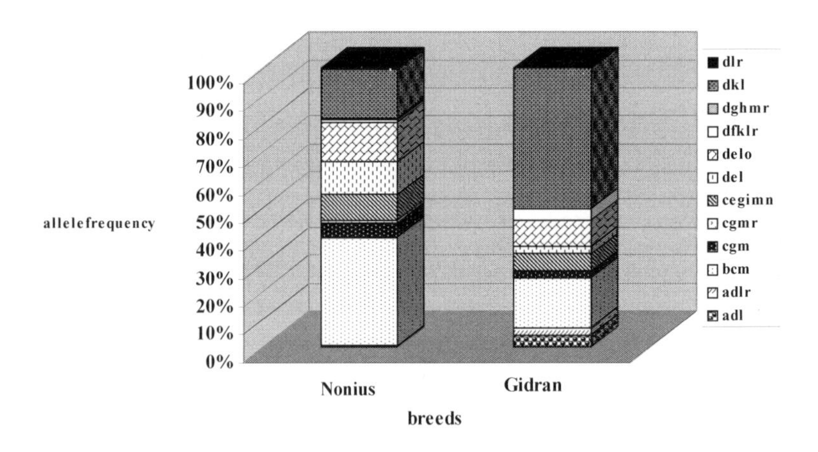

Figure 3. Distribution of D blood group alleles.

Biochemical polimorphic systems

The Tf^D and Tf^{F2} transferrin alleles were dominant in both breeds (Nonius 0.2714 and 0.3839, Gidran 0,2727 and 0,3485 respectively). The exclusive alleles observed only in one breed were Tf^E (0,1393), (Tf^G 0,0036) for the Nonius and Tf^{F3} for the Gidran breed.

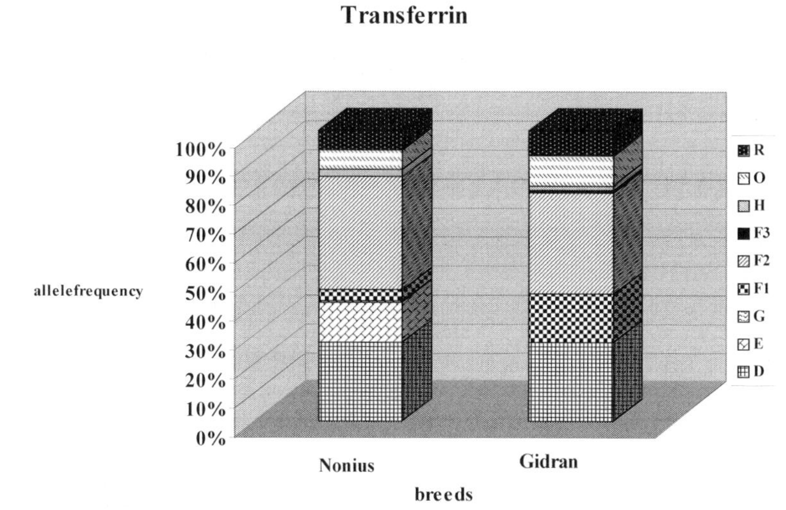

Figure 4. Frequencies of transferrin alleles in Nonius and Gidran

No difference could be observed in albumin, GC and A1B systems. The existing alleles and their frequencies were similar in both breeds. The "B" albumin, the "F" GC and the "K" alelles were dominant.

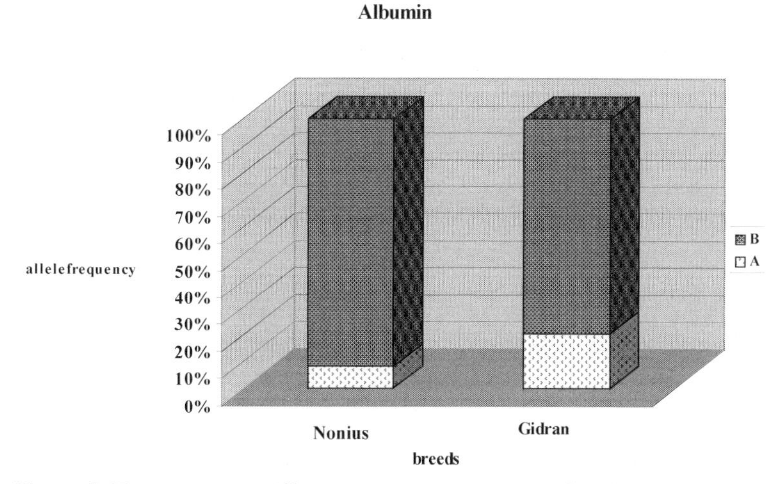

Figure 5. Frequencies in Albumin system in Nonius and Gidran.

Four alleles were detected in esterase system in both breeds with dominant "I" allele. In Nonius, however high frequency of "F" allele was observed (0,3178).

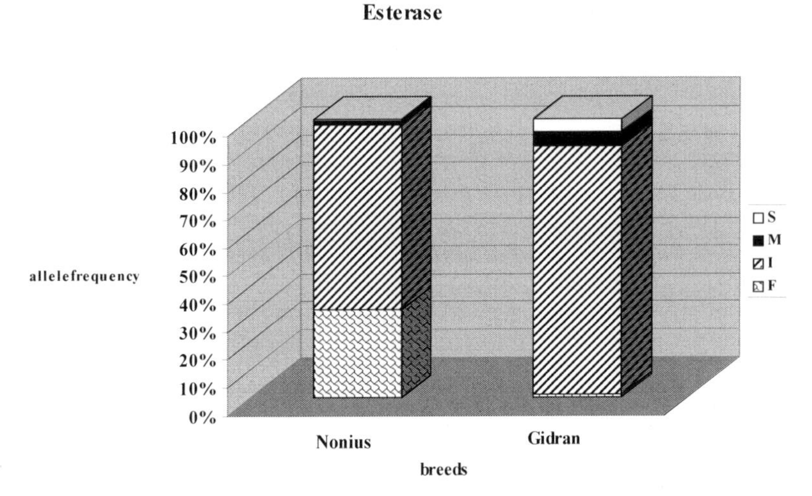

Figure 6. Distribution of esterase alleles.

Results of DNA investigations

In **AHT4** microsatellite 8 alleles were found in both breeds. Exclusive alleles for Nonius were AHT4-P and AHT4-Q for Gidran AHT4-L and AHT4-N. Dominant alleles were in Nonius AHT4-H (0,293) in Gidran AHT4-J (0,3406).

In **AHT5** microsatellite 5 alleles (J, K, M, N, O) were found in both breeds with different frequencies. Dominant alleles were in Nonius AHT5-J (0,4850) in Gidran AHT5-K (0,3678).

The frequency of **ASB2** alleles were high in both breeds (Nonius 12, Gidran 10). The dominant allele was ASB2-K. Exclusive alleles were in Nonius ASB2-C, ASB2-D, ASB2-H and ASB2-J, in Gidran ASB2-O and ASB2-R.

In Nonius 12, in Gidran 7 **HMS2** microsatellite alleles were found. In the later the HMS2-S allele, in Nonius HMS2-I,

HMS2-O, HMS2-P, HMS2-Q and HMS2-T alelles were observed, which could not be seen in the other breed.

From **HMS3** microsatellite 8 alleles (I, M, N, O, P, Q, R, S), from **HTG6** 8 (G, I, J, K, M, O, P, R), from **HMS7** 7(J, K, L, M, N, O, P) could be observed with different frequencies.

In Gidran 6 alleles, in Nonius 7 alleles from **HMS6** microsatellite were isolated. In Gidran HMS6-N was not observed, in Nonius its frequency was low (0,004). The dominant allele was HMS6-P (Nonius 0,3380, Gidran 0,33238).

From **HTG10** microsatellite 10 alleles were demonstrated in Gidran and 11 in Nonius breeds. The dominant alelle was HTG10-O in both (Gidran 0,3191, Nonius 0,2610). In Nonius HTG10-J and HTG10-N alleles could be found , in Gidran HTG10-S as well.

Seven **HTG4** microatelite alleles were observed in both investigated breeds. The frequency was different, the dominant allele was the same HTG4-M (Nonius 0,6840, Gidran 0,7813).

In the Nonius samples in **HTG7** microsatellite only 4 alleles (K, M, N, O) in Gidran 6 alleles (J, K, M, N, O, P) were observed. The dominant allele was the same HTG7-O in Nonius (0.544) and Gidran (0,617).

In **VHL20** microsatellite 8 alleles (I, L, M, N, O, P, Q, R) were isolated in Nonius and 7 alleles (I, L, M, N, P, Q, R) in Gidran breeds. In Nonius the VHL20-M (0,2180) and in Gidran the VHL20-I (0,3740) alleles were the dominant ones.

The alleles and allele frequencies (12 microsatellites) of the two investigated breeds are different. In some cases different microsatellites were found in the samples of the investigated breeds (ASB2, HMS2). In the case of some microsatellites (HMS3, HTG6, HMS7) the number of alleles was the same, but the frequencies were different in both breeds.

Based upon the frequency of alleles the Gidran breed proved to be more homogeneous than the Nonius. This statement corresponds well with the pedigree analysis of the breeds in question. In some cases the common origin of these two breeds was expressed in the similar alelle frequencies (Figure 7 and Figure 8.).

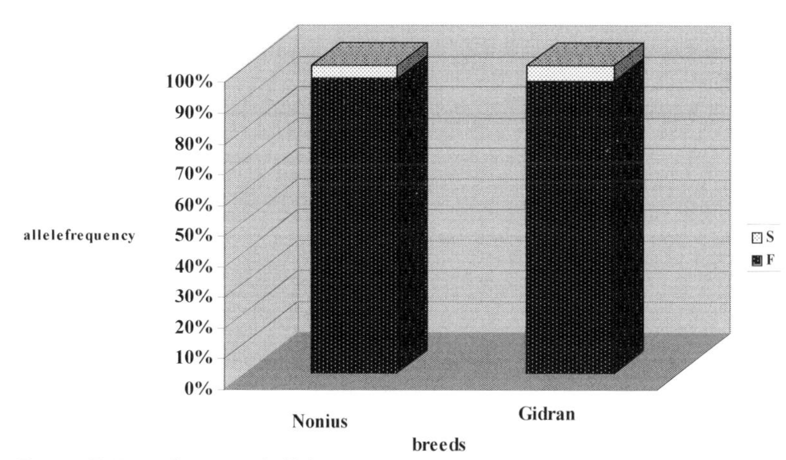

Figure 7. Distribution of alleles in GC system.

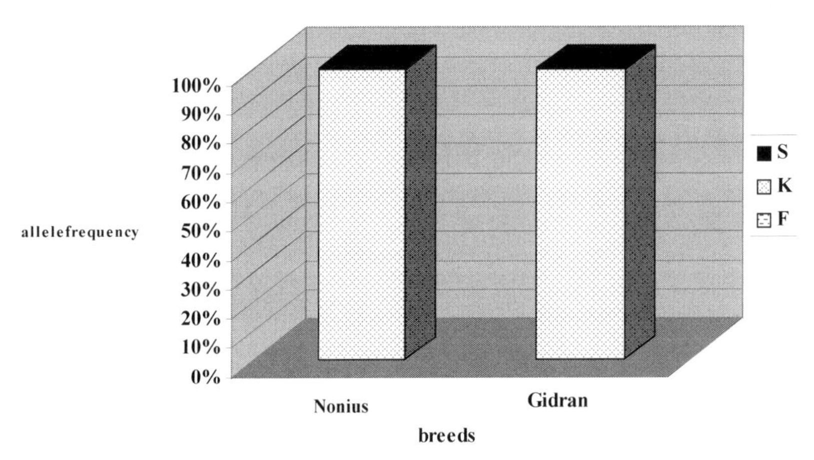

Figure 8. Distribution of alleles of A1B system.

The comparison of Nonius, Gidran and English Thoroughbred

Based upon the allele numbers and frequency of "D" blood group, and Transferrin systems it could be stated, that Gidran is more similar to the Thoroughbred breed than Nonius, corresponding well to the history, the pedigree analysis and conformation. of the breeds.

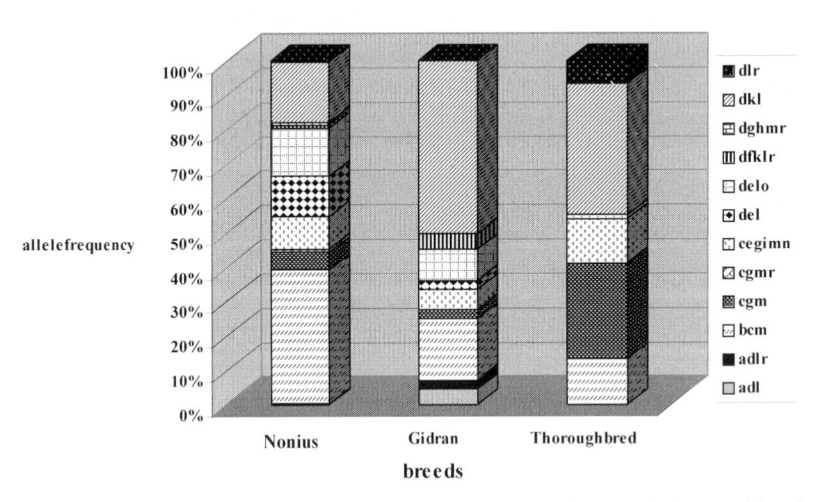

Figure 9. Comparison of D blood group of Nonius, Gidran and Thoroughbred.

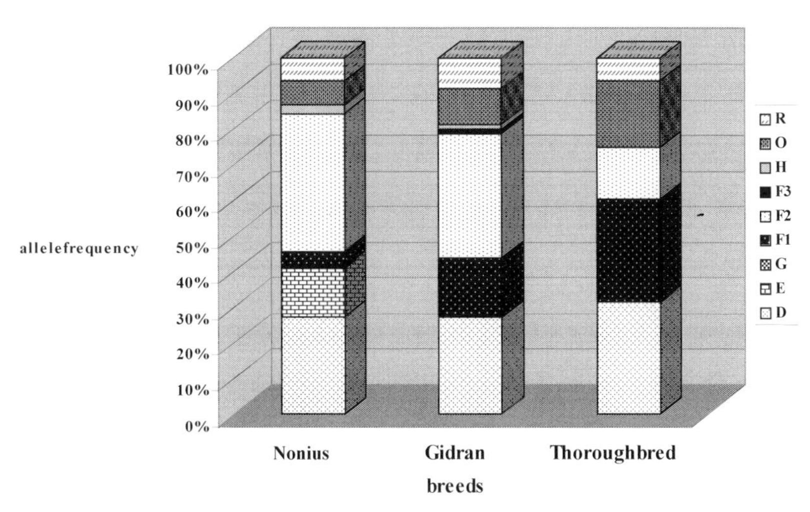

Figure 10. Comparison of Transferrin of Nonius, Gidran and Thoroughbred.

In AHT5 microsatellite 5-5 alleles (J, K, M, N, O) occurred in the investigated breeds and their frequency was more similar in Thoroughbreds and Gidrans than in Nonius.

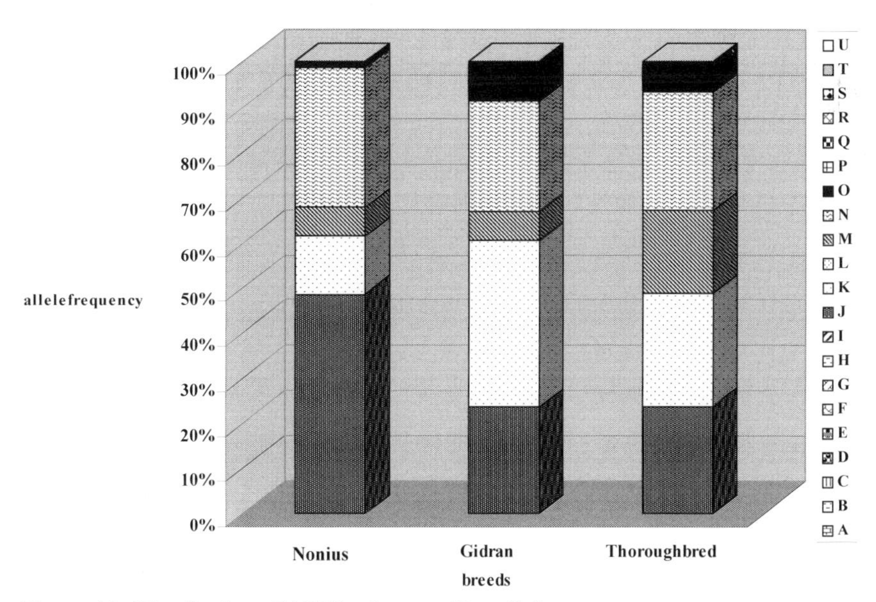

Figure 11. Distribution of AHT5 microsatellite alleles.

The same in HTG6 microsatellite 8 alleles (G, I, J, K, M, O, P, R) occured in Nonius and Gidran samples. I, K and P alleles in Nonius and Gidran were observed in low frequency, however in Thoroughbred it could not be detected. The frequency of observed alleles in Gidran and Thoroughbred were more similar compared to Nonius. It corresponds well to the history of the breeds.

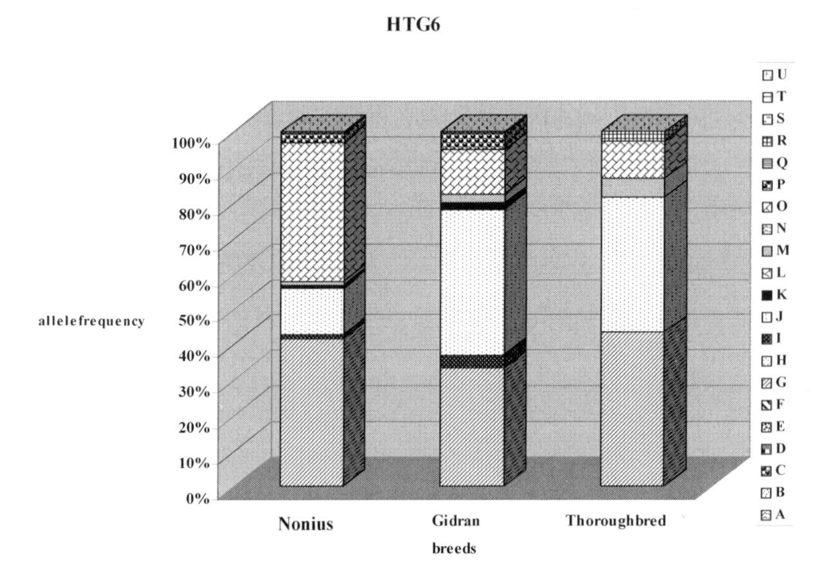

Figure 12. Distribution of HTG6 microsatellite alleles.

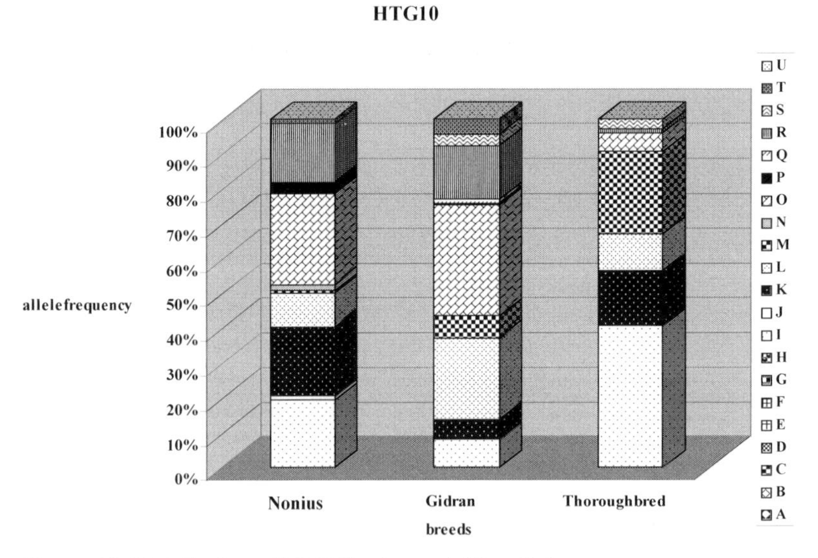

Figure 13. Distribution of HTG10 microsatellite alleles.

Based upon the microsatellite investigations the conclusion can be drawn that the alleles of Thoroughbred horses could be observed in both breeds (Nonius and Gidran). The number of alleles were higher compared to the Thoroughbred breed. In the case of polymorphic alleles (ASB2, HMS2, HTG10) many of them could be observed and their frequency was different. From the aspect of the other microsatellite alleles Nonius, Gidran and English Thoroughbred were more similar.

Conclusions

It appears relevant that immunogenetics and molecular genetics increased our knowledge about the genetic structure of the breeds bred in Mezőhegyes much more than two centuries ago. The frequency of alleles of Gidran breed has shown it to be more homogeneous than the Nonius. This statement corresponds well with the well known history of the breeds in question. In some cases the common origin of these two breeds was expressed in the similar alelle frequencies.

The frequency of observed alleles in Gidran and Thoroughbred were more similar compared to Nonius.

Furioso-North Star, the Mezőhegyes Halfbred breed will be involved later in the project.

Estimation of genetic distance between breeds, lines and families is important for breeding strategies and long term decisions. Within the breeding goal of preservation the presence of rare alleles is a new point, which can be taken into consideration among others in everyday pratice as well.

References

Andersson, L., 1985. The estimation of blood group gene frequencies a note on the allocation methods. Anim. Blood. Groups. Biochem. Genet. 16. 1-7.p.

Bán, B., Cs. Józsa and A. Gyurman, 2002. Thoroughbred and Trotter Blood Group and DNA allele Frequency in Hungary. XXVIII. International Conference on Animal Genetics D003., Göttingen.

Binns, M.M., N.G. Holmes, A. Holliman and A.M. Scott, 1995. The identification of polymorphic microsatellite loci in the horse and their use in Thoroughbred parenatage testing. British Veterinary Journal 151. 9-15.p.

Bodó, I., 2000. Ed. Living heritage Agroinform Budapest 126.p.

Bowling, A.T., 1996. Horse Genetics CAB International, Wallingford.

Bowling, A.T., M.L. Eggleston-Scott, G. Byrns, R.S. Clark, S. Dileanis and E. Wictum, 1997. Validation of microdsatellite markers for routine horse parentage testing. Animal Genetics 28. 247-252.p.

Dohy, J., I. Bodó and O. Mátay, 1982. Efforts for maintaining rare non commercial native breeds in Hungary. EAAP Leningrad G.1.6.8.

Kakoi, H., T. Tozaki, S. Mashima and K. Hirota, 1998. Evaluation of new microsatellite markers for horse parentage testing. Abstracts. Animal Genetics 29.15.

Marklund, S., H. Ellegren, S. Eriksson, K. Sandberg and L. Andersson,1994. Parentage testing and linkage analysis in the horse using a set of highly polymorphic microsatellites. Animal Genetics 25. 19-23.p.

Nei, M. 1972. Genetic distance between populations. Am. Nat. 106. 283-292.p.

Ócsag, I. 1984. A nóniusz (The Nonius) Mezőgazdasági Kiadó. Budapest.

Pataki, B., 2000. Nonius. In Living heritage. Ed. I Bodó. Agroinform Budapest 10-11.p.

Pataki, B., 2000. Gidran In Living heritage. Ed. I Bodó. Agroinform Budapest 12-13.p.

Pirchner, F. 1983. Population genetics in animal breeding Freeman Company San Francisco.

Van Haeringen, H., A.T. Bowling, M.L. Stott, J.A. Lenstra and K.A. Zwaagstra, 1994. A highly polymorphic horse microsatellite locus VHL20. Animal Genmetics 25 207.

Wrangel, C.G., 1893. Ungarns Pferdezucht I.,II. Stuttgart.

Genetic diversity of the Akhal-Teke horse breed in Turkmenistan based on microsatellite analysis

A. Szontagh[1], B. Bán[2], I. Bodó[3], E.G. Cothran[4], W. Hecker[1], Cs. Józsa[2], Á. Major[5]

[1]University of Kaposvár, Department of Cattle Breeding, H-7400 Guba Sándor u. 40., Hungary
[2]National Institute for Agricultural Quality Control, Laboratory of Immunogenetics, H-1024 Budapest, Keleti Károly u. 24., Hungary
[3]University of Debrecen, Department of Animal Breeding and Nutrition, H-4032 Debrecen, Böszörményi út 138., Hungary
[4]University of Kentucky, Department of Veterinary Science, Lexington, KY 40546, USA
[5]Roland Eötvös University, Dep. of Genetics, H-1117, Pázmány Péter sétány 1/c, Hungary

Abstract

A sample of the Turkmenian stock of the ancient Akhal Teke horse breed, indigenous in Turkmenistan and regarded to be a genetic resource, were genotyped for 12 DNA microsatellites. To place results in context, DNA samples of the following breeds were also analyzed: Standardbred, Thoroughbred, Turkoman horses from Iran and Akhal Teke populations from the USA and Iran. The number of alleles per locus and the effective number of alleles per locus reveal that the breed has a relatively high allelic diversity. The average genetic diversity measured as expected heterozygosity (H_e) was 0.7. The mean F_{IS} value, used for estimating the inbreeding, came to 0.053 showing a negligible deficit of heterozygotes. Despite of the separation and long history of the Akhal Teke horses, compared to other breeds its genetic diversity appears not to have reduced. The data gained from the analysis of DNA samples of non-Turkmenian Akhal Teke populations included in the study also supports this conclusion.

1. Introduction

The Akhal-Teke horse breed, indigenous in Central Asia in the area of Turkmenistan (Figure 1) in the Akhal Oasis and named after it, can be considered to be one of the oldest horse breeds of the World.

According to the local tradition, its history counts several thousands of years. The Akhal Teke was generically known as the Turkoman until the end of the 19th century when Russia conquered the Turkomans and incorporated them into her Empire. However, in the Iranian area, inhabited by the Turkmens, this ancient breed still bears the same name. The Turkoman horse has been always famous for its legendary performance and conformation (Figure 2) Akhal-Teke stallion from the Nyazov stud, Ashgabat, Turkmenistan. /Photo: A. Szontagh/)

As several authors have pointed out, the Turkoman horse might have contributed to the development of the English Thoroughbred and it also influenced the Trakehnen breed (Oettingen, 1908; Belonogov, 1955; Hecker, 1972). Hence, its effect on the World's horse breeding is enormous and a number of breeds that belong to the English part-bred - among them our traditional Hungarian breeds, - could be genetically related to the Turkoman horse.

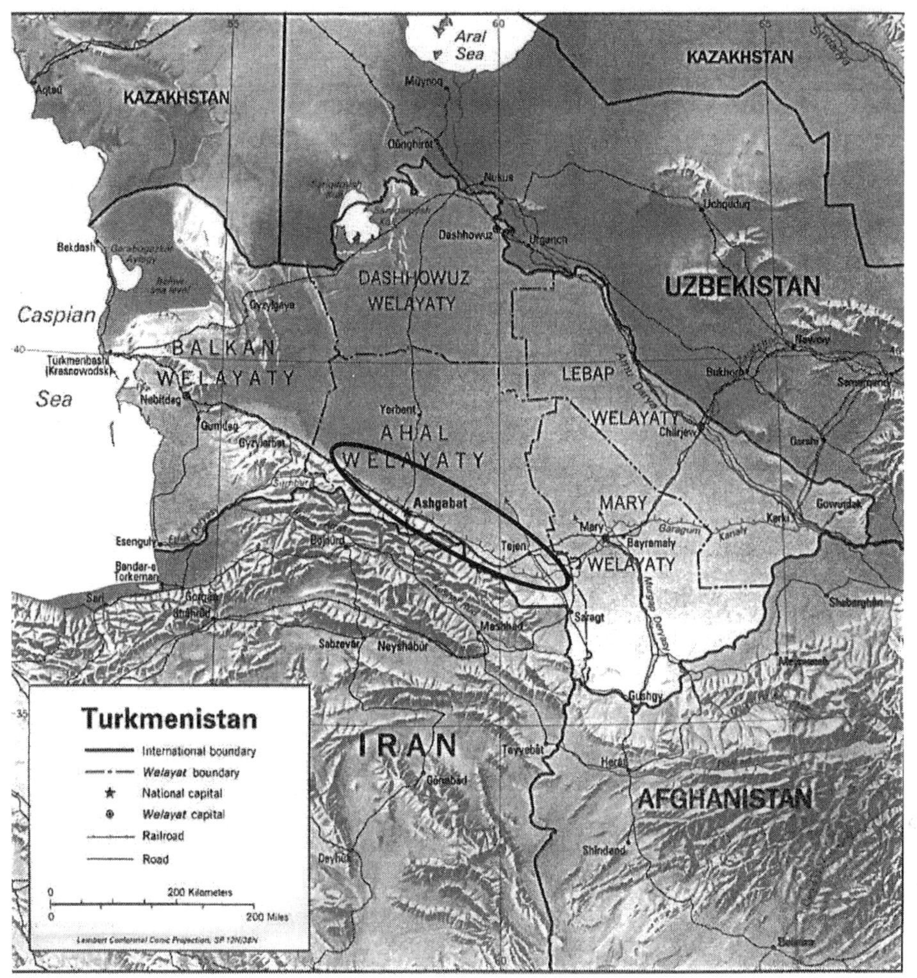

Figure 1.

An explicitly Hungarian-related aspect is worth mentioning. The Hungarian conquerors' horses (originating from the East) might have had impacts from the genetic center of Turkoman horses before the 9th century. During the centuries after the Conquest, as a result of military events or trade, horses from similar Central-Asian origin also appeared, and were involved in the Hungarian horse breeding up to the end of the 18th century (Jankovich, 1970).

The outstanding historic and cultural importance of the Akhal-Teke and its role in the development of today's horse breeds predestinate it to be a genetic resource of outstanding importance (Bodó, 1992), which provided the ground for the investigation of its genetic diversity. The Akhal-Teke, considering the size of the population, does not belong to the most endangered horse breeds of the World; however, all relevant available official FAO data originate from the time before Turkmenistan's independence. Special agricultural circumstances and poor competitiveness have led to a sharp decline in the purebred population. On the other hand, there are breeder societies not only in Russia but in the West as well (www.fao.org/dad-is).

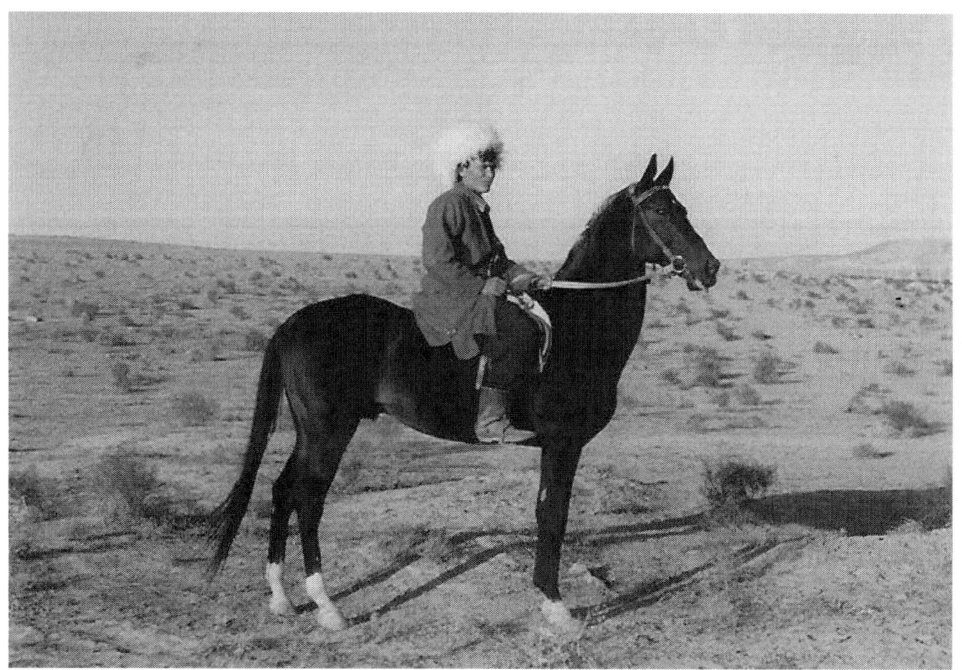

Figure 2.

Even the literature of the Soviet era mentioned a distinct characteristic of the Akhal-Teke in relation to the blood group systems (Dimitriev and Ernst, 1989.) and some later publications have made genetic data based on mSat-research as reference-breed available (i.a. Horín *et al*., 1998.) These data, however, do not characterize the indigenous stock in Turkmenistan, whereas the present research is trying to fill this gap. This work is restricted to publishing the first results of a larger project that is to involve further investigations.

In addition to the Turkmenian (AT T) material, we also incorporated data on Akhal-Teke horses from the USA (AT US, n=58 individuals) and Iran (AT I, n=19) and on the Turkoman from northern Iran (TURK, n=17). This latter is considered to be the closest relative to the Akhal-Teke breed in the research. To put the research in a wider context, Hungarian Thoroughbred (THB, n=38) and Standardbred (STB, n=50) populations were also included in the research as reference breeds.

2. Materials and methods

2.1. Sampling

Sampling was performed in southern Turkmenistan in the area of Akhal Oasis (Figure 1: Map of Turkmenistan indicating the Akhal-area. /Source of map: http://www.lib.utexas.edu/maps/turkmenistan) during autumn, 1998. Hair samples were taken from 48 individuals (29 stallions and 19 mares) of 9 populations from a broad geographical range. Horses were randomly chosen but being aware of the pedigrees, the closely related animals (parent-offspring, sibling) were excluded from the analysis.

2.2. DNA extraction, PCR amplification, microsatellite markers

The DNA was extracted from the hair-bulbs by using a 5% Chelex solution. After having extracted the DNA, the fragments were amplified on a GeneAmp PCR System 9700. Applied Biosystems StockMarks® Kit for Horses was used in the procedure according to the StockMarks® Protocol. The samples were analysed on an ABI PRISMTM 310 DNA Sequencer. The evaluation was carried out with GenotyperTM software run on a Macintosh computer.

The individuals were genotyped at 12 dinucleotide repeat microsatellite loci, namely VHL20 (van Haeringen *et al*., 1994), HTG4, HTG6 (Ellegreen *et al*., 1992), AHT4, AHT5 (Binns *et al*., 1995), HMS7, HMS6, HMS3, HMS2 (Guerin *et al*., 1994), HTG10, HTG7 (Marklund *et al*., 1994), and ASB2 (Breen *et al*., 1997).

2.3.Computations

The number of alleles was calculated by direct count. The observed and the expected heterozygosities (Ho, He) and the deviations from the Hardy-Weinberg equilibrium were obtained using Arlequin Version 2.000 software (Schneider, 2000). The effective number of alleles (Ne) was calculated as follows: Ne = 1/(1-He) (Kimura and Crow, 1964), the mean F_{IS} value, used for estimating the level of inbreeding, was calculated as F_{IS} = 1-Ho/He (Nei and Chesser, 1983).

3. Results and discussion

Table 1 summarizes the number of alleles (N), the mean number of alleles (MNA), the effective number of alleles (Ne) per loci, the heterozygosity (Ho and He) and the F_{IS} values. A total of 73 alleles was detected across the 12 loci, with locus VHL20 showing the highest number of alleles. The number of alleles, which can such be considered high, ranged from 4 to 9. The STB and the Turkoman approach the allele number of the Turkmenian Akhal-Tekes, whereas the Iranian and US populations exceed it. The MNA values show the relatively high allelic diversity of the investigated population, and this is most remarkably manifested in the US Akhal-Teke and Turkoman horses. The effective numbers of alleles (Ne) indicate the alleles' real impact, because the more equal the allele frequencies are, the more they contribute to the absolute number of the detected alleles. In this case the three Akhal-Teke and the Turkoman populations show a notable superiority (4.03, 4.03, 4.20 and 4.52, respectively) compared to the values below 4 in the Standardbred and Thoroughbred (3.66 and 3.53). Considering the MNA and Ne values of the table we cannot count with the decrease of allelic diversity with the Akhal-Teke breed.

As expected, the detected allelic number increases with the sample size, so the US sample shows high allele values. The high values of the Iranian populations are also notable.

The genetic diversity measured as the expected heterozygosity (He) resulted in 0.703 and ranged between 0.410 (HTG4) and 0.870 (ASB2), and the observed heterozygosity resulted in 0.664 and ranged between 0.396 and 0.917 (on the same loci). This level cannot be considered as being reduced, and the US Akhal-Teke and the two Iranian populations show even greater heterozygosity. The narrower range of the reference breeds (STB: He 0.524-0.864, Ho 0.575-0.820; THB: He 0.612-0.843, Ho 0.553-0.868) also shows a considerable genetic variance for the studied population. Considering the World-average value (0.694), which has been calculated from several breeds (Horín, *et al*. 1998), a decrease in heterozygosity can only be detected at the Standardbred.

Table 1. Numbers of alleles, observed, expected heterozygosities and the F_{IS} values.

	N	MNA	Ne	Ho	He	F_{IS}
AT T	73	6,1	4,03	0,664	0,703	0,053
AT US	91	7,6	4,03	0,655	0,727	0,100
AT I	70	5,8	4,20	0,728	0,725	-0,005
TURK	80	6,7	4,52	0,773	0,757	-0,025
THB	63	5,3	3,66	0,678	0,705	0,036
STB	72	6,0	3,53	0,651	0,676	0,036

The F_{IS} value, used for estimating the inbreeding level, is 0.053 in the investigated population, which reflects only a minor lack of heterozygosity. The increased inbreeding (F_{IS}=0.100) of the US population could be the consequence of its isolation.

The results of the test for the Hardy-Weinberg equilibrium, reveal a significant (P=0.05) deficit of heterozygotes only at one locus (HMS3) of the Turkmenian Akhal-Tekes. All 12 loci of both Iranian populations are in equilibrium. Four loci in the US Akhal-Teke (ASB2, HMS3, HTG10, HTG6), 4 loci of the STB (AHT4, ASB2, HMS3, HTG10) and 2 loci of the THB (ASB2, HTG10) are in disequilibrium. In the case of the Iranian horses – taking into account the small size of the sample – this shows the stability of these populations.

Table 2. Hardy-Weinberg equilibrium.[1]

Loci	AT T			AT I			TURK			AT US			THB			STB		
	Ho	He	P	Ho	He	P	Ho	He	P	Ho	He	P	Ho	He	P	Ho	He	P
AHT4	0.500	0.663	0.104	0.737	0.848	0.522	0.706	0.702	0.983	0.586	0.695	0.084	0.711	0.689	0.255	0.680	0.728	0.002
AHT5	0.660	0.630	0.172	0.684	0.728	0.551	0.571	0.606	0.800	0.655	0.731	0.067	0.857	0.788	0.558	0.776	0.750	0.452
ASB2	0.917	0.871	0.790	0.947	0.841	0.818	0.706	0.786	0.248	0.785	0.866	0.034	0.618	0.844	0.001	0.676	0.864	0.002
HMS2	0.756	0.844	0.195	0.737	0.787	0.678	0.823	0.813	0.346	0.768	0.799	0.145	0.600	0.654	0.707	0.575	0.651	0.241
HMS3	0.646	0.792	0.036	0.789	0.774	0.926	0.882	0.788	0.879	0.741	0.768	0.047	0.763	0.679	0.289	0.660	0.700	0.039
HMS6	0.771	0.742	0.304	0.842	0.757	0.874	0.765	0.764	0.741	0.596	0.736	0.094	0.711	0.656	0.692	0.820	0.794	0.235
HMS7	0.702	0.753	0.830	0.789	0.762	0.904	0.765	0.756	0.968	0.759	0.775	0.566	0.811	0.789	0.954	0.838	0.587	0.612
HTG10	0.646	0.686	0.386	0.684	0.642	0.967	0.706	0.844	0.765	0.667	0.762	0.010	0.541	0.772	0.000	0.469	0.524	0.034
HTG4	0.396	0.410	0.616	0.579	0.549	1.000	0.824	0.688	0.465	0.552	0.567	0.164	0.553	0.612	0.645	0.720	0.735	0.118
HTG6	0.708	0.687	0.125	0.632	0.755	0.150	0.706	0.790	0.428	0.466	0.631	0.000	0.553	0.661	0.054	0.540	0.542	0.948
HTG7	0.521	0.534	0.159	0.421	0.431	1.000	0.824	0.668	0.548	0.569	0.615	0.158	0.553	0.614	0.357	0.460	0.502	0.242
VHL20	0.750	0.825	0.419	0.895	0.822	0.396	1.000	0.872	0.831	0.719	0.777	0.536	0.868	0.704	0.142	0.800	0.736	0.765

[1]Ho, He and p values in bold, where the locus is not in equilibrium (P=0.05).

Besides inbreeding, the locus may also be under selection that can result in a lack of heterozygosity. Therefore, in the case of the Turkmenian horses we can count on a more pronounced selection intensity in the whole population caused by the centralized, state-coordinated breeding in the previous decades in the Soviet Union as compared to Iran. This is also indicated by the larger F_{IS} value. The results of the test with the US population, in correlation with the F_{IS} values, also show a greater lack of heterozygosity. The putative presence of null alleles (non-amplifying alleles) should be mentioned here since they can also lead to a distorted Hardy-Weinberg equilibrium. In addition, the lack of heterozygosity could derive from the substructure of the population that may lead to Wahlund's effect.

4. Conclusions

During the analysis of the sample from the indigenous stock that can be considered as the most representative one, we have come to the conclusion that the genetic diversity in the Akhal-Teke horse breed in Turkmenistan appears not to be reduced. Compared with the reference breeds, the allelic diversity is especially significant, and the deviation from the Hardy-Weinberg equilibrium is also unlikely. The results of the Turkoman and the Iranian Akhal-Teke horses also reinforce this conclusion, but the isolated US Akhal-Teke do not unambiguously underpin this. This means that keeping this genetic resource without exhausting its genetic variance could be successful in its Central Asian homeland.

5. Acknowledgements

The authors would like to express Mr. András Vutskics (Europharma Ltd.), the Brendon Ltd. and the wife of the late marquis Dr. Roger Csáky-Pallavicini their gratitude for their generous financial contribution without which this work could not have been completed. We also thank Dr. Erzsébet Takács Head of the Laboratory of Immunogenetics, National Institute for Agricultural Quality Control for her great help in the preparation of this study.

6. References

Belonogov, M.M., 1955. Osnovnie polozenia po plemennoj rabote s ahaltekinskoj parodoj losadej. Academy of Sciences of the Turkmenian SSR, Ashgabat.

Binns, M.M., N.G. Holmes, A. Holliman and A.M. Scott, 1995. The identification of polymorphic microsatellite loci in the horse and their use in Thoroughbred parentage testing. Brit. Vet. J. 151, 9-15.

Bodó, I., 1992. A Global Review of the Genetic Resources of Equidae. FAO, Animal Production and Health Paper. 104, 215 – 226.

Breen, M., G. Lindgren, M.M. Binns, J. Norman, Z. Irvin, K. Bell, K. Sandberg and H. Ellegren, 1997. Genetical and physical assignment of equine microsatellites: first integration of anchored markers in horse genome mapping. Mammal Genome. 8, 267-273.

Dmitriev, N.G. and L.K. Ernst, 1989. Animal Genetic Resources of the USSR. FAO. Rome. An. Prod. Health Paper. 65, 259.

Ellegren, H., M. Johansson, K. Sandberg and L. Andersson, 1992: Cloning of highly polymorphic microsatellites in the horse. Animal Genetics. 23, 133-142.

Guérin, G., M. Bertaud and Y. Amigues, 1994: Characterization of seven new horse microsatellites: HMS1, HMS2, HMS3, HMS5, HMS6, HMS7 and HMS8. Animal Genetics. 25, 62.

Hecker, W., 1974. Az üllői fakótenyészet tenyésztési célkitűzései (The Breeding Aims of the Dam Stud in Üllő). Lovassport - lótenyésztés. 19/5, 23-29.

Horín, P., E.G. Cothran, K. Trtková, E. Marti, V. Glasnák, P. Henney, M. Vysocil and S. Lazary, 1998. Polymorphism of Old Kladruber horses, a surviving but endangered baroque breed. European Journal of Immunogenetics. 25, 357-363.

Jankovich, M., 1970. A magyar ló. (The Hungarian Horse) Agrártörténeti szemle. 12./3-4, 253-257.

Kimura, M. and J.F. Crow, 1964. The number of alleles that can be maintained in a finite population. Genetics. 49, 725-738.

Marklund, S., H. Ellegren, S. Eriksson, K. Sandberg and L. Andersson, 1994. Parentage testing and linkage analysis in the horse using a set of highly polymorphic microsatellites. Animal Genetics. 25, 19-23.

Nei, M. and R.K. Chesser, 1983. Estimation of fixation indices and gene diversities. Annals of Human Genetics. 47, 253-259.

von Oettingen, B., 1908. Zuht des edlen Pferdes. Verlagbuchhandlung Paul Parey, Berlin, 8.

Schneider S., D. Roessli and L. Excoffier, 2000. Arlequin: A Software for Population Genetics Data Analysis, Ver. 2.000. Genetics and Biometry Laboratory, Department of Anthropology, University of Geneva, Geneva.

Van Haeringen, H., A.T. Bowling, M. Stott, J.A. Lenstra and K.A. Zwaagstra, 1994. A highly polymorphic horse microsatellite locus: VHL20. Animal Genetics. 25, 207.

Rare horse breeds in Northern Europe

M.T. Saastamoinen[1] and M. Mäenpää[2]
[1]Agrifood Research Finland, Equine Research, Varsanojantie 63, 32100 Ypäjä, Finland
[2]Suomen Hippos, Tulkinkuja 3, 02650 Espoo, Finland

Summary

The Nordic Gene Bank for Farm Animals keeps a list of rare horse breeds in the Nordic and Baltic countries. Those on the list are local breeds, mainly coldbloods, small horses or ponies. The breeds are well adapted to the cold climate and to other circumstances in their countries of origin. Many have a common origin and are closely related to each other. These horse breeds have previously played an important part in farm and forest work as well as in transport. After mechanisation of farming and transport, the number of individuals in the breeds has declined and their role has shifted to modern uses like riding, driving and trekking. The small population size in many breeds has led to inbreeding, and efforts have been made to restrict this through breeding planning. A lot of work has been done at the national and inter-Nordic levels to preserve these rare horse breeds and the valuable gene material they carry.

Keywords: biodiversity, horse breeding, conservation of horse breeds

Introduction

Altogether 17 horse breeds are listed on the Nordic Gene Bank for Farm Animals' (Nordisk Genbank Husdyr, NGH) list of rare breeds, although some can be considered as the same breed. Fourteen of them have "conservation" status. The breeds are from the Nordic countries (Denmark, Finland, Norway, Sweden) and the Baltic countries (Estonia, Latvia, Lithuania). In addition, there are three breeds that can be regarded as rare but are missing from the list: the Frederiksborg Horse (Denmark), the Faer Island Pony (Faer Islands/Denmark) and the Mezen Horse (North-West Russia). Furthermore, the Icelandic Horse, known all over the world, is a national breed but is not considered a rare breed. The breeds are shown in Table 1.

The rare horse breeds are mainly coldbloods, small horses or ponies. Many of them have common origins and are closely related to each other. The number of horses in each breed has decreased dramatically after World War II as a result of mechanised farming and transportation. For example, the Finnhorse population has diminished since the 1950s from 400 000 individuals to 20 000, and the Estonian Native Horse from 16 000 to 500. On the other hand, some breeds have gained wide popularity outside their home countries, and their numbers have increased. The best example is the Icelandic Horse. Some countries do not register the number of horses in each breed, and in some populations only the number of horses registered in studbooks are given. Thus, the true status of all breeds is not known.

The breed data presented here are based mainly on NGH's www pages, Hendricks (1995) and SOU (2000), as well as on information obtained from national breeding organisations.

Table 1. National horse breeds in Northern Europe

Breed	Country	Population size
Doele Horse (C)	Norway	4000
Estonian Draught (C)	Estonia	70-80
Estonian Native Horse (P)	Estonia	900
Faer Island Pony (P)	Faer Islands/Denmark	47
Finnhorse (C)	Finland	20000
Fjord Horse (C, S)	Norway	6000
Frederiksborg Horse (W)	Denmark	?
Gotland Russ (P)	Sweden	8000
Jutland (C)	Denmark	?
Latvian Warmblood (W)	Latvia	17000
Lithuanian Heavy Draught (C)	Lithuania	400
Mezen Horse (C)	Russia	1000
Nordland (C, S)	Norway	2300
North-Swedish Horse (C)	Sweden	4500
+ Norwegian Trotter (C)	Norway	11000
+ Swedish Trotter (C)	Sweden	8000
Swedish Ardennes (C)	Sweden	4500
Toric (C)	Estonia	650
Zemaitukai (S)	Lithuania	300
Icelandic Horse (S)	Iceland	74000

C = coldblood, S = small horse, P = pony, W= warmblood
Sources www.nordgen.org, Hendricks (1995), national horse breeding organisations

Rare breeds in different countries

The Nordic countries

There are two local horse breeds in Denmark – the Jutland and the Frederiksborg – but only the Jutland is on the list of rare horse breeds. In addition, there is a local pony breed on the Faer Islands, which belong to Denmark.

The Frederiksborg Horse is the oldest native horse breed in Denmark, dating back to the 16th century. The breed was very famous during the 17th – 19th centuries, and horses were exported to many countries to form and improve other breeds. The Frederiksborg was used both as a riding horse, a carriage horse and a military horse. The breed is nowadays crossed with lighter warmblooded breeds. To be entered in the studbook, a horse shall have less than 50% genes from other breeds. The number of individuals is not registered, but there are about 160 – 300 active mares (Staun, 1999, Köhler, 2004). The Knabstrup is a descendant, a lighter version of the Frederiksborg Horse. The number of mares in breeding is less than 200.

The Jutland is a draught horse breed originating from 1850. The ancient origins of the breed are not known, but breeders have used breeds like the Suffolk, Cleveland Bay and French Ardennais in forming and upgrading the breed. The studbook is closed, and the number of individuals has declined during the years, leading to a high degree of inbreeding. The number of active mares is only around 200 (Staun, 1999, Köhler, 2004). One problem in the breed is a high frequency of side bones, and selecting against them is difficult because of the small population size. The Faer Island Pony is a very rare breed, with less than 50 individuals (Leivsson, 2004). The breed originates from horses that arrived along with settlers from Scandinavia and the British Isles, and is closely related to the Icelandic Horse. Nowadays the breed is used for pleasure riding.

The Finnhorse is the only local breed in Finland. Like some other northern breeds, it may have its origins in Northern forest horses (< Tarpan), but it has been developed by crossing various breeds over the centuries – including the Frisian, several European and Baltic breeds (16th – 17th centuries), Swedish horses (18th century), as well as the Orlov and other Russian breeds, the Norfolk Trotter and the Swedish Ardennes (19th century). Pure breeding was begun in 1895, and the studbook was closed in 1907. No crossings have been allowed since then. The Finnhorse was used in the early 20th century to create and improve some Baltic and Russian horse breeds. The breed was previously used for farm work, but today its main uses are in trotting and riding sports as well as in agritourism and small-scale forest work. The Finnhorse also has a small horse (pony) type. Today the number of horses has risen to 20 000 from a record low population in the early 1980s. About 2000 mares are inseminated yearly.

Norway has three local horse breeds. The Nordland Horse (Lyngen Horse) has the smallest number of individuals, about 2300. The horses are of pony size. This breed originates from Northern forest horses and has been developed from small breeds that used to live in the country's northern regions. Organised breeding was begun in the 1930s, and a thoroughbred stallion was used in breeding (Olsen et al., 2004). The pony-type Finnhorse was also used in breeding in the 1960s. The main use of the Nordland Horse was previously in agriculture, but today it is used for hobby riding as well as logging. Again, because of the limited active population size, inbreeding is a problem.

The Fjord is a very old horse breed, which is believed to be related to the Przewalski Horse. It has been estimated that the Fjord Horse migrated to Norway about 4000 years ago and was domesticated 2000 years ago. The breed has influenced the development of most West-European heavy draught horse breeds. The Fjord is a small horse formerly employed in agriculture and forestry, and nowadays used mainly for pleasure riding, driving and forest work. This breed has been exported to many European countries as well as to the US and Canada.

The Doele Horse is a result of crossing native breeds (partly descended from the Frisian) with Danish breeds and, e.g., the Norfolk and Holstein breeds. Pure breeding was started in 1874. Because of trotting sports and the introduction of the totalisator game in 1928, the breed was separated into two types. Since then the population of the heavy Doele Horse has decreased as a result of farm work mechanisation. Trotting-type Doele Horses were developed into the Norwegian Coldblood Trotter, which is considered the same breed as the Swedish Coldblood Trotter. These two populations (Norwegian and Swedish Coldblood Trotters) have exchanged genetic material for about half a century, and common breeding evaluation has been carried out since 1994. There is strong inbreeding among the heavy type Doele Horse, and this has led to reduced fertility. The heavy Doele Horse and the North-Swedish Horse are so closely related that they are accepted in each other's studbooks. The Norwegian Coldblood Trotter is not allowed to breed with the Doele Horse (Olsen et al., 2004).

The North-Swedish Horse is of the same origin as the Doele Horse, and about 100 years old as a breed. There are two types of horses in this breed: a draught horse and a trotter (Swedish Coldblood Trotter). The Swedish Ardennes was developed by crossing lighter Swedish country horses with imported Ardennais Horses in the late 19th century. Belgian Draught were also used. There has been a dramatic decline in population size: in 1948, there were 26 500 served mares, whereas today the number of individuals in the breed is only about 4500 altogether. The Swedish Ardennes has been used in creating the Estonian Draught Horse. The number of mares covered is about 620 for the North-Swedish Horse and 570 for the Swedish Ardennes (Witt et al., 2004).

The only national native horse breed in Sweden is the Gotland Russ (Gotland Pony). The breed is descended from Northern forest horses. It is also related to the Konik and the Hucul. It is possible that several other breeds also have genetic links to the Gotland Russ. The breed's ancestors may have lived on the Isle of Gotland since the Stone Age. The breed is used mainly for riding but also for pony trotting in Sweden and Finland. The number of covered mares is about 560 yearly (Witt et al., 2004).

The Icelandic horse is an old native breed, aged more than 1000 years. It is of Celtic origin and was created using Shetland, Highland and Connemara Ponies – the last one of which, in turn, is descended from the Fjord Horse. It is not a rare breed, as the total number of individuals around the world is about 200 000. In Iceland its population has increased to 74 000 over the past 200 years. The Icelandic Horse is purebred and isolated: no crossings with other breeds have been made in 1000 years. It has five gaits (the fifth one is called the toelt), and the main weight in breeding selection is on the gaits. All horse colours are found in the breed. Modern methods are actively used in breeding evaluation: a selection index has been applied from 1950 onwards and the BLUP method since 1979.

The Baltic countries

The Estonian Native Horse (Klepper) is a pony-size horse. It is one of the last survivors of the horse breeds belonging to the Northern forest horse group, and thus has common ancestors with other Baltic and Russian native breeds. It may also be related to the Gotland Russ (< Konik, Hucul < Tarpan). The breed was formerly used in farming and for transport. During the Soviet era the original type of the Estonian Native Horse almost disappeared because of the need for larger horses for heavy farm work. Estonian Native Horses were therefore crossed with heavier breeds, including the Finnhorse and the Fjord Horse. The breed was also used in creating the other Estonian breeds: the Toric and the Estonian Draught. Before World War II the population size of the Estonian Native Horse was 12 000 – 16 000. Nowadays there are only about 900 individuals, but their number continues to grow. There is no inbreeding depression in the breed. There is an efficient breed conservation programme ongoing in Estonia, connected to environment protection and tourism projects. The number of foals born per year is more than 150.

The Toric Horse (Tori) is a relatively new breed developed for farm work and transport in the late 19th and early 20th century. It was formed by crossing the Estonian native horse with a variety of breeds, e.g. the Frisian, Hackney, Norfolk and Arabian. Nowadays Toric Horses are crossed with lighter warmblooded breeds, such as the Hannoverian and Holstein. The number of the old-type heavy Toric Horses is about 600-700 individuals, and only about 10 foals of that type are born yearly, against to appr. 100 cross-bred Toric foals. The Estonian Draught Horse was recognised as a breed in 1953. It was also developed from the Estonian Native Horse by crossing it with the Swedish Ardennes. There are only 70-80 individuals left in this breed, and only about 10 foals are born per year.

The Latvian Warmblood was developed by crossing the Latvian Native Horse with Lithuanian and Estonian Native Horses in the 18th century. The Latvian Native Horse was probably related to the Doele Horse. Later, at the beginning of the 19th century, the use of the Oldenburg, Hannover, Groeningen and Holstein breeds in breeding was started. Also the Ardennes and Frisian have been widely used. The Latvian Warmblood includes heavier and lighter types of horses. Since World War II, the breed has been improved by crossing with the Hannover, Oldenburg and Danish Warmblood to develop the breed as a sport horse.

The Zemaitukai (Zhmud, Zhemaichu, Zhumdka) is a native Lithuanian breed which is related to the Estonian Native Horse (< Northern forest horses) and the Konik. It is believed to be descended from the Tarpan. This is one of the oldest breeds in Europe and is known from the 6th and 7th centuries. The breed has been influenced by other breeds over the centuries, e.g. by Polish breeds and Arabs. The total number of individuals in the breed is low, only about 160. The breed has also a lighter and taller type of horse, the Modern-type Zemaitukai. It was created late in the 19th century by crossing Zemaitukais with the Orlov and the North-Swedish Horse. The population size is about 150.

The Lithuanian Heavy Draught has been developed from the Zemaitukai by crossing it with the Swedish Ardennes and the Finnhorse. The breed was confirmed in 1963. Its stock was at its largest in 1964, with 64 000 individuals. Today, however, the population is only about 400.

North-West Russia

In Arkhangelsk region in the North-West part of Russia, there is a native breed called the Mezen Horse. Its population size is about 1000 individuals, but the number of productive mares is only 64. The Mezen Horse is a small draught horse, descended from the Northern forest horse and related to, e.g., the Estonian Native Horse and the Zemaitukai. Finnhorses and Estonian Native Horses have been used in breeding the Mezen, but during the last fifty years the breed has been bred pure. It is well adapted to hard northern climatic conditions and to insect bites in the summer. The horse is used for farm work and transport, and it is especially valuable in the autumn slush and in deep winter snow. The Arkhangelsk Scientific-Research Institute of Agriculture has taken measures to protect the breed since 1993.

The Viatka Horse is another native Russian horse breed in the Kirov and Western Perm regions and in Udmurtia. It is of the same origin as the Estonian Native Horse and the Zemaitukai, and of about same size. The breed is almost extinct: there are only about 1000 pure Viatka Horses left (Hendricks, 1995).

Breed characteristics and use

Many of the local breeds are adapted to the often harsh northern climatic and other conditions as well as to low-nutrient feeds and diets with low concentrate (grain) levels. Studies with Icelandic horses, e.g., show that the breed is well adapted to highly fibrous feeds (Sverrisdottir et al., 1993). The last intestine (where fibres are mainly digested) of the Icelandic horse comprises a larger part of the digestive tract than other horse breeds. Its carbohydrate metabolism is also very efficient, resulting in the accumulation of fats and sensitivity to laminatis. These characteristics can be suggested to belong to some other northern breeds as well. Saastamoinen (1993) found differences in energy expenditure between Finnhorses and warmblooded horses. In addition, Icelandic Horses have been found to adapt to lower Se-levels (Vervuert et al., 2004) and to different Cu- and Zn-levels compared to those used in other European countries (Vervuert et al., 2004; Stark et al., 2001). If these aspects are not taken into account when various native breeds are exported to other countries and different circumstances, the horses may encounter health problems. The Icelandic Horse, e.g., has proved very sensitive to insect bites.

Earlier, the primary importance of the breeds was in farm work, forest work and transportation. Nowadays these horses are mostly used for pleasure riding, trekking and driving. Still, some breeds (e.g. Finnhorse, Fjord, Jutland, North-Swedish horse) are especially suitable for forestry work and continue to be used for this purpose. Some are mainly employed in trotting sports (Finnhorse as well as Norwegian and Swedish Coldblood Trotters). In any case, the new purposes are essentially important with respect to the conservation of the breeds and of the valuable genes they carry.

Local breeds also have a specific and increasingly important role in preserving landscapes and biodiversity in the countryside. They are significant in developing new, horse-related activities like agritourism. Farmers are actively involved in this activity. Moreover, the influence of many native breeds in creating new breeds and upgrading others has been considerable.

Problem of inbreeding

Because of the very small population size of some breeds, it is difficult to avoid inbreeding – and this may result in very strong inbreeding. In addition, many of the populations are closed. The generation intervals between sire and son and sire and daughter have increased, e.g. being 11 – 12 years for the Finnhorse and the Norwegian Coldblood Trotter (Immonen, 1992; Oikarinen, 2002; Klemetsdal, 1993a). A situation like this calls for control and restriction of the inbreeding rate.

In many breeds, the rate of inbreeding has accelerated during recent decades; in the Finnhorse, e.g., the inbreeding coefficient has doubled over the past 10 years (Oikarinen, 2002). The strongest inbreeding has been observed for the Jutland, which has an inbreeding coefficient close to 15% (Table 2). Strong inbreeding exists also in the Nordland and Doele Horses (Vangen, 1983; Olsen & Klemetsdal, 2003, Olsen *et al.*, 2004). For the Nordland, the average inbreeding coefficient used to be even higher, 15 – 19%, but has declined in the last decades. In contrast, the inbreeding coefficient for the Doele has increased. Finnhorses (Immonen, 1992; Oikarinen, 2002) and Fjord Horses (Vangen, 1983), on the other hand, exhibit a low inbreeding rate.

Table 2. Inbreeding coefficients for some breeds.

Breed	Inbreeding coefficient (F)
Doele horse	12.0
Nordland Horse	12.0
Jutland	14.7
Norwegian Trotter	5.5-6.0
North-Swedish Trotter	4.5
Finnhorse	3.0-3.5
Fjord Horse	3.3

Sources Immonen (1992), Klemetsdal (1993a), Staun (1999), Olsen & Klemetsdal (2003), Olsen et al. (2004), national breeding organisations

The most common way of reducing the rate of inbreeding is to introduce new genes into the breed by crossing. This has been done in the Jutland, e.g., by crossing with the Suffolk, and in the Estonian Native Horse and the Nordland Horse by crossing with the Finnhorse. Klemetsdal (1993b) introduced a sire selection strategy to reduce inbreeding in Swedish and Norwegian Coldblood Trotters. Additionally, there is a PC programme to avoid close matings, developed by the Danish Institute of Agricultural Science (DIAS) and financed by the NGH (www.nordgen.org, www.agrsci.dk). This software, called the EVA (Evolutionary Algorithm for Mate Selection), has also been demonstrated in Finland for the Finnhorse. The EVA can be used for mating plans, since it calculates the optimal genetic contribution of the parents to maximise the genetic trend and restrict inbreeding.

Work for conservation

The Nordic Gene Bank for Farm Animals, NGH, plays a major role in the efforts to protect rare breeds and conserve their valuable genes. In addition, horse organisations and breeding associations in many countries are actively promoting the use and conservation of native and rare breeds.

The NGH has working groups for various animal species – also one for horses. The members of the group come from Denmark, Finland, Iceland, Norway and Sweden. Their task is to create guidelines for ensuring the preservation of the genetic resources of the horse in the Nordic countries. Although the NGH is a Nordic organisation, it maintains co-operation ties with the Baltic countries and also with Russia, especially in regard to the northern regions of the country.

The NGH will publish a manual on how to manage the protection of the breeds in each country, with respect to population size and structure, etc. The organisation has carried out projects related to horses, e.g. “Genetic variation in Doele horses and Nordlands” (Olsen & Klemetsdal, 2003) and will start a project on the diversity of horse populations together with the Baltic countries and Western Russia. Further, as noted, the EVA software for the preparation of mating plans was financed by the NGH. Networking and meetings are also an important part of the organisation’s annual activities.

In addition, the Nordic countries have their own national strategies for preserving the native and rare breeds and their gene resources, including breeding plans. Breeding organisations and governments are responsible for this work. In North-West Russia, e.g., the Arkhangelisk Scientific Research Institute has set up a stud farm for the Mezen Horse and implemented research projects promoting the conservation of the breed.

Research and training in forestry work with horses has recently been carried out in the Nordic countries. This supports the use and breeding of rare horse breeds and, thereby, their conservation. In some local and EU-funded projects, horses graze natural pastures for landscape preservation. The protection of the Estonian Native Horse has been connected in Estonia to a nature conservation programme and agritourism. In Finland, EU subsidies for native breeds are paid to Finnhorse breeders.

References

Hendricks, B.L., 1995. International Encyclopedia of Horse Breeds. University of Oklahoma Press, Norman and London. 1st ed. 478 p.

Immonen, T., 1992. Sukusiitosaste ja sukupolven välinen aika suomenhevospopulaatiossa [Inbreeding and generation interval in Finnhorses]. M. Sci. Thesis. University of Helsinki. Helsinki. 51 p.
Klemetsdal, G., 1993a. Demographic parameters and inbreeding in the Norwegian trotter. Acta Agricultural Science, Sect. A Animal Science 43: 1-8.
Klemetsdal, G., 1993b. Sire selection strategies in North-Swedish and Norwegian trotters. Paper, 44th EAAP meeting. 20 p.
Köhler, L., 2004. Danish horses. NGH-NYTT, 3/2004, p. 9.
Leivsson, T., 2004. Faer Island pony. NGH-NYTT, 3/2004, p. 7.
Oikarinen, H., 2002. Muutokset suomenhevospopulaation rakenteessa [Changes in the structure of Finnhorse population]. Paper, Seminar in animal breeding, University of Helsinki. 6 p.
Olsen, H.F. and G. Klemetsdal, 2003. Genetic variation in two local Norwegian horse breeds. Report of NGH-project. 3 p.
Olsen, H.F., G. Klemetsdal, J. Ruane and T. Helfjord, 2004. Genetic variation and pedigree structure in two endangered Norwegian horse breeds. Paper, 55th EAAP Ann. Meeting, 18 p.
Saastamoinen, M., 1993. Feed, energy and protein intakes of horses – A review of Finnish feeding trials. Agricultural Science in Finland 2: 25-32.
SOU, 2000. En svensk hästpolitik. Betänkande av Hästpolitiska utredningen. SOU 2000: 109. Stockholm 2000. 261 p.
Staun, H., 1999. The actual breeding policy within Danish draught horse breeds. In: Proceedings of international seminar on working horses: Use of horses in forestry and agriculture. Breeding of working horses. Maijala, K. (ed). p. 119-124.
Stark, G., B. Schneider and M. Gemeiner, 2001. Zinc and copper plasma levels in Icelandic horses with Culicoides hypersensitivity. Equine Veterinary Journal 33 (5): 506-509.
Sverrisdottir, K., I. Sveinsson and G.Ö. Gudmundsson, 1993. The digestive tract of the Icelandic horse. Paper, EAAP cosponsored International Symposium Horse Breeding and Production in Cold Climatic Conditions, Reykjavik 1993. 6 p.
Vangen, O., 1983. The use of relationship matrices to avoid inbreeding in small populations. Zeitschrift für Tierzucht und Züchtungsbiologie, 100: 48-54.
Vervuert, I., M. Coenen and S. Braun, 2004. Fütterungpraxis von Islandpferden in Island und nach Import in Deutschland unter besonderer Berücksichtigung der Selenversorgung – 1. Mitteilung. Pfredeheilkunde 20 (1): 23-29.
Witt, P., D-A. Danielsson and Z. Kurowska, 2004. Horse breeding in Sweden. NGH-NYTT, 3/2004, p. 8.

Use of probabilities of gene origin to describe genetic varation in two endangered Norwegian horse breeds

H.F. Olsen[1], *G. Klemetsdal*[1], *J. Ruane*[1,2] *and T. Helfjord*[3]

[1]*Department of Animal and Aquacultural Sciences, Norwegian University of Life Sciences, P.O. Box 5003, N-1432 Ås, Norway*
[2]*Current address: Food and Agriculture Organization of the United Nations (FAO), Viale delle Terme di Caracalla, 00100 Rome, Italy*
[3]*Norwegian Equine Centre, Starum, N-2850 Lena, Norway*

Abstract

The Norwegian Døle horse and the Nordland/Lyngen horse are two small, endangered populations where artificial selection is exercised. As this leads to reduced effective population size and accelerated genetic drift, which further leads to loss of genetic variation and possible accumulation of recessives, the genetic variance in these two breeds was examined by use of probabilities of gene origin, in addition to the rate of inbreeding. Key parameters such as inbreeding coefficients, effective population size, effective number of founders, effective number of ancestors and effective number of founder genomes were calculated. The level of inbreeding in the two breeds was about 12%, and when considering the last generations, the effective population sizes were 158 in the Døle horse, and 62 in the Nordland/Lyngen horse. The sensitivity of calculating a reliable inbreeding rate, and consequently the effective population size, was shown by regressing individual inbreeding coefficients on year of birth of horses. By using a complementary approach, using the probabilities of gene origin, the calculations revealed that there was great skewness in the genetic contributions to the reference populations (horses born 1990-1998), and that the genetic variation in the populations is likely to be greatly reduced. This highlights the need for careful planning of the future breeding of these two breeds.

Keywords: breed conservation, effective population size, probability of gene origin

Introduction

Norway has, despite its relatively wealth of domestic animal genetic resources (Ruane, 2000), several breeds that are threatened by extinction. Most of these breeds are traditional Norwegian domestic breeds, where the challenge consists in providing for public awareness, surveying the populations and ensuring that the breeds are managed in a sustainable way so that problems of inbreeding and loss of genetic variation are minimised.

The Norwegian Døle horse and the Nordland/Lyngen horse are local breeds with a long tradition. These breeds have originally been used as working horses in farming and forestry, but have today another range of use as a natural consequence of the industrial revolution. It is well known that these breeds have a high level of inbreeding, but there is no recent description of its range and consequence. Artificial selection is also carried out in these small populations, which reduces the effective population size. In an already small population this accelerates the genetic drift, in which allele frequencies at a locus change at random from one generation to the next, leading to the eventual fixation of alleles and reduction of additive genetic variation. The genotype frequencies will also be affected, where the frequencies of homozygotes increase and recessives accumulate in the population, a phenomenon known as inbreeding depression.

The former reports on these breeds' state have not revealed any alarming results (Vangen, 1983), but still there was a need for a new evaluation of the situation, based on the possibility of using complementary methods of describing the genetic variation, such as probabilities of gene origin. The objective of this study was to look closer at the methodology used to describe genetic variation, by calculating various parameters directly relevant for breed conservation efforts in two endangered Norwegian horse breeds.

Material and methods

Data were received from the Norwegian Equine Centre in autumn 1999, with 30,712 registered animals of the Døle and 1,983 registered animals of the Nordland/Lyngen. The birth-years of the Døle-population stretched from 1846 to 1998, whereas the Nordland/Lyngen-population contained horses born from 1906 to 1998. Initially, the files were edited to remove obvious errors, and it was checked that all sires and dams also had been assigned an ID-number. At the end of this procedure, the total number of records generated for the two breeds were 31,142 in Døle and 1,987 in Nordland/Lyngen. Then, all the ID-numbers were renumbered. The reference populations were defined as horses born between 1990 and 1998, with founders defined as horses with unknown parents. When an animal had only one parent known (half-founder), the unknown parent was considered as a founder (Boichard *et al.*, 1997).

Effective population size

Several measures can be used to describe the genetic variation in a population. To quantify the rate of genetic drift, the rate of inbreeding is most frequently used (Boichard *et al.*, 1997). Individual inbreeding coefficients, from the renumbered pedigree, were calculated using the Quaas-Henderson algorithm (Quaas, 1976; Henderson, 1976). The effective population size is defined as the number of individuals in an idealised population which would give rise to the same inbreeding rate (ΔF) as observed in the real population (Falconer & Mackay, 1996). The effective population size was computed as:

$$\frac{1}{N_e} = 2\frac{F_t - F_{t-1}}{1 - F_{t-1}} = 2\Delta F \quad (1)$$

where F_t is the average coefficient of inbreeding in the defined reference population, in generation t, and F_{t-1} is the average inbreeding coefficient of parents of these individuals, in generation t-1.

To show the complexity of calculating a reliable rate of F and consequently the effective population size, an approximate value of ΔF was calculated by regressing individual inbreeding coefficients on year of birth of horses. Simple linear regression was estimated for three periods, 1990-1998, 1980-1998 and 1970-1998, to examine the trend in rate of inbreeding. The effective population size was approximated by:

$$\frac{1}{N_e} = 2\Delta F_y L \quad (2)$$

where ΔF_y is the simple linear regression estimate of yearly rate of inbreeding and L is the calculated generation interval between parents and progeny, for the corresponding time period.

A complementary approach, which is more robust to incomplete data, is to analyse the probabilities of gene origin, i.e. the effective number of founders (f_e), effective number of ancestors (f_a) and effective number of founder genomes (f_g) (Boichard *et al.*, 1997).

Effective number of founders

Effective number of founders was defined as the number of equally contributing founders that would produce the same genetic diversity as in the reference population under study (Lacy, 1989; Rochambeau *et al.*, 1989):

$$f_e = 1 \Big/ \sum_{k=1}^{f} q_k^2 \qquad (3)$$

where q_k is the genetic contribution of founder k to the population's gene pool. If each founder contributes the same, the effective number of founders equals the actual number of founders, measuring the preservation of the genetic diversity from the founders to the present population. In any other situation, the effective number will be smaller than the actual number of founders. The approach ignores potential bottlenecks in the pedigree (Boichard *et al.*, 1997).

To carry out these calculations all ancestors of the animals in the reference populations were traced back to the founders in an accumulation procedure, individual-by-individual, also to reveal the completeness of the data. Each animal in the reference population was listed with its respective ancestors per generation backwards (Example 1). The table has to be read from the bottom and up, and each animal in the reference population is in generation 1, whereas their parents are in generation 2, their grandparents are in generation 3 and so on.

Example 1. Result file after the accumulation procedure, relevant for one animal in Family 2 in Boichard et al. *(1997).*

ID-number	Sire	Dam	Generation	Founder contribution
0004	0000	0000	3	0.25
0005	0000	0000	3	0.25
0004	0000	0000	3	0.25
0005	0000	0000	3	0.25
0002	0005	0004	2	-
0003	0005	0004	2	-
0001	0003	0002	1	-

By means of the generation number (*g*) attached to each animal, the contribution from founder k, by animal, was calculated as $1/(2^{g-1})$. Corresponding contribution from half-founders was calculated as $1/(2^g)$. Notice that within animal the founder contributions sum to 1 (Example 1). Now, say that the reference population was made up of another fullsib of individual 1. To derive the founder contribution to the two (all) animals in the reference population, we first summarized the contributions per founder k, then divided by the number of animals in the reference population, resulting in q_k (½ for individual 4 and 5, respectively) (Formula (4)). In essence, the approach assumes that an allele, randomly sampled, has a 0.5 probability of originating from any of its parents. Boichard *et al.* (1997) used the same rule to derive an algorithm which only necessitates one run through the data from the youngest to the oldest by initiating a vector of contributions (q_0) with 1 for animals in the reference population, otherwise zero. Example 2 shows q values when processing individual-by-individual (e.g. q_1, when processed individual 1):

if sire (i) is known then q(sire(i)) = q(sire(i)) + 0.5*q(i),

if dam (i) is known then q(dam(i)) = q(dam(i)) + 0.5*q(i);

Example 2. Pedigree input to Boichard et al. (1997)'s algorithm calculating founder contributions.

ID-number	Sire	Dam	q_0	q_1	q_2	q_3
0001	0003	0002	1	1	1	1
0002	0005	0004	0	0.5	0.5	0.5
0003	0005	0004	0	0.5	0.5	0.5
0004	0000	0000	0	0	0.25	0.5
0005	0000	0000	0	0	0.25	0.5

The vector q must be divided by the number of individuals in the reference population, so that the founder contributions sum to 1.

Effective number of ancestors

The effective number of ancestors is the minimum number of ancestors (which may or may not be founders) required to explain the complete genetic diversity of the population under study (Boichard *et al.*, 1997):

$$f_a = 1 \Big/ \sum_{k=1}^{f} p_k^2 \qquad (4)$$

where:

$$p_k = q_k \left(1 - \sum_{i=1}^{n-1} a_i\right) \qquad (5)$$

and p_k is the marginal contribution of ancestor k to the population's gene pool, which is q_k adjusted for the genetic contribution a_i from the n-1 already selected ancestors. Initially, it is logical to determine the largest contributing ancestor as the one having the largest q-value. When determined, the contributions taken out by that animal should not be assigned to more remote ancestors, taken account of by eliminating its pedigree information, leaving the animal as a "pseudo founder". The animal's descendants also need to get their contributions adjusted for the contribution from this pseudo founder; leading to calculations of marginal contributions, i.e. the contribution not explained by other ancestors. The marginal contributions from all ancestors will sum to 1.

For this task we used a pedigree file where all the animals ever registered in the population were listed with information on ID-number (re-numbered in descending order, from the youngest to the oldest), sire and dam. We used Boichard *et al.* (1997)'s algorithm, as explained. A vector q was assigned with 1 to the animals in the reference population (horses born 1990-1998), whereas all the others were assigned with 0. In the first iteration the ancestor with the highest marginal contribution ($p_X = q_X$) was determined. In iteration two, X's sire and dam information was deleted, before q-values again were calculated.

Furthermore, sorted from the oldest to the youngest, a vector a was initiated with 1 for X, and with 0 otherwise. Running through the data once, assigning:

$a(i) = a(i) + 0.5*a(sire(i))$, if sire(i) is known,

$a(i) = a(i) + 0.5*a(dam(i))$ if dam(i) is known,

keeping track of contributions from pseudo founders to descendants. The animal's marginal contribution (p_k) was calculated by the use of q_k and a_i. Then the highest marginal contributing ancestor in iteration two was picked out, and the procedure above was repeated. The q's and the a's were updated each iteration. This procedure continued until all the ancestors had been assigned their marginal contribution to the reference population. Finally, the effective number of ancestors could be calculated. For further details about the original algorithm, see Boichard *et al.* (1997).

In the Nordland/Lyngen all ancestors with a non-zero contribution to the reference population were determined. In the Døle we stopped the procedure with the 100 highest contributing ancestors, as these individuals covered more than 97% of the contribution to the reference population. The effective number of ancestors accounts for potential bottlenecks, but still the probability of gene loss by drift needs to be considered.

Effective number of founder genomes

To account for loss of genetic variability by genetic drift, Lacy (1989, 1995) and Ballou & Lacy (1995) proposed the concept of effective number of founder genomes, or founder genome equivalent. This measures the number of founder genes that are maintained in the population for a given locus, and how balanced their frequency is. Originally, this parameter was calculated as a probability (Lacy, 1989), or by gene dropping analysis (MacCluer *et al.*, 1986). Alternatively, Lacy (1995) proposed to stay with a definition of the founder genome equivalent as half the inverse of average coancestry, or average mean kinship, in generation t:

$$f_g = \frac{1}{2\bar{f}_t} \tag{6}$$

This has been supported, especially from a practical point of view, by Caballero & Toro (2000) and Zechner *et al.* (2002).

The coancestry of two animals is identical with the inbreeding coefficient of their progeny if they were mated (Falconer & Mackay, 1996). To derive the average coancestry for the reference population, we calculated the inbreeding coefficients of "dummy progenies" from imaginary matings between all the animals in the reference population, independent of gender and including selfing, resulting in n(n+1)/2 records, where n is the number of animals in the reference population. The average coancestry was calculated as the average coefficient of inbreeding of the dummy offspring.

Results

The reference populations, defined as horses born between 1990 and 1998, consisted of 1,535 horses in the Døle and 1,050 in the Nordland/Lyngen (Table 1). The total number of registered animals of the Døle was 31,142 animals, of which 11,757 animals (38%) were founders. In the Nordland/Lyngen, the number of registered animals was 1,987, of which 73 animals were founders (4%). Six generations backwards from the reference population, both breeds had a pedigree completeness of more than 95%, while in generation 10 the completeness had decreased to 74% in the Døle and only 20% in the Nordland/Lyngen (Table 1).

Table 1. Number of animals in the reference population and parameters describing the pedigree of the reference population; in the Døle and in the Nordland/Lyngen.

		Døle	N/L
# animals in the reference population		1,535	1,050
# animals in the pedigree (total)		31,142	1,987
# founders in the pedigree		11,757	73
% known ancestors in generation	2	99.97	99.95
	6	95.39	98.91
	10	73.58	19.77

Figure 1 shows the evolution of the level of inbreeding in the two breeds over the past 100 years. The average inbreeding coefficient in the last decade was about 12% in both breeds, but they have developed somewhat differently. In the Døle the average inbreeding coefficient increased to about 7% in the 1940's, after which it fell significantly, before rising again towards the end of the 1970's. For the Nordland/Lyngen, the average inbreeding coefficient has been high for a longer period.

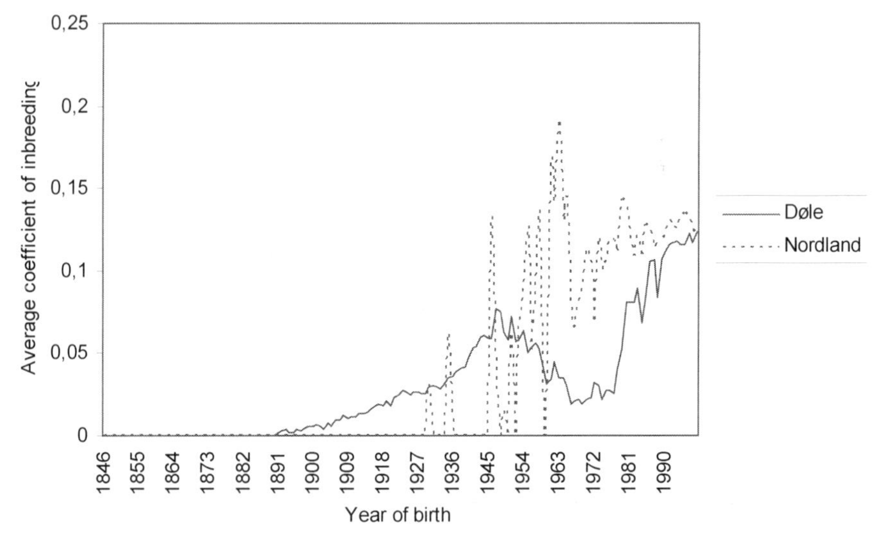

Figure 1. Average coefficient of inbreeding per year of birth; in the Døle and in the Nordland/Lyngen.

The average coefficient of inbreeding of the reference populations was 11.75% in the Døle, as a result of an increase of 0.28% the last generation, and 12.77% in the Nordland/Lyngen, increasing 0.71% over the last generation (Table 2). The effective population size was calculated using formula (1) as 158 in the Døle, and 62 in the Nordland/Lyngen. When using regression and formula (2), the results differed somewhat for the effective population size. In the first time period, 1990-1998, the results were not significant, but by including longer time periods a lower estimate was calculated for N_e in the Døle, and a higher estimate for N_e in the Nordland/Lyngen (Table 2).

Table 2. Calculated parameters of inbreeding and rate of inbreeding through effective population size, describing genetic diversity of the reference population; in the Døle and in the Nordland/Lyngen.

		Døle			N/L		
Average coefficient of inbreeding (F_t)		0.1175			0.1277		
Increase of average coefficient of inbreeding, last generation, (F_t-F_{t-1})		0.0028			0.0071		
Effective population size (N_e)		158			62		
		β_1	L	N_e	β_1	L	N_e
Estimated N_e[1] by regression:	1990-98	0.00096[2]	9.1	57	-0.00008[2]	8.6	∞[1]
	1980-98	0.00264[3]	9.2	21	0.00051[3]	8.5	116[2]
	1970-98	0.00420[3]	9.7	12	0.00075[3]	8.6	78[3]

[1] $1/N_e = 2\Delta F_y L$, from annual rate of inbreeding (ΔF_y) approximated by simple regression of individual inbreeding coefficients on year of birth of horses (β_1), and generation interval between parents and progeny (L).

[2] $P \geq 0.05$.

[3] $P < 0.01$.

In the pedigrees of the reference populations, the number of founders was 770 in the Døle and 49 in the Nordland/Lyngen (Table 3). The results from the probabilities of gene origin, the effective number of founders, the effective number of ancestors and the effective number of founder genomes, were 48, 12 and 5.4 respectively in the Døle, and 14, 7 and 3.7 respectively in the Nordland/Lyngen.

Table 3. Calculated parameters of gene origin, describing genetic diversity of the reference population; in the Døle and in the Nordland/Lyngen.

	Døle	N/L
Number of founders (f)	770	49
Effective number of founders (f_e)	48	14
Effective number of ancestors (f_a)	12	7
Effective number of founder genomes (f_g)	5.4	3.7

Discussion

Both breeds have a large pedigree completeness of the reference populations, although in Døle the number of founders is quite large. When the first herd-book for the Døle was published in 1902, they had systematized an already existing and accepted practise, and there was little work done in tracking all the ancestors far back. In the Nordland/Lyngen, the systematic registration of the breed started after the Second World War, as an attempt to save the breed from extinction. At this point, there were very few individuals alive, so the registration work was quite easy, and this can explain the large pedigree completeness in the first 6 generations backwards from the reference population of this breed.

The development of the level of inbreeding in the two breeds has been quite different. The Døle had a peak in the level of inbreeding around 1950. At this point there was discussion about possible inbreeding depression in the Døle, especially in connection to reduced fertility (Gaustad, 1951). As an effort to deal with this rising problem, stallions of the Norwegian cold-blooded trotter were allowed to breed in the Døle, for the first time in 1953 (Gaustad, 1953), as the Norwegian cold-blooded trotters have the same genetic origin as the Døle (Fridrichsen, 1961). As a result, the level of inbreeding decreased until the 1970's, when the breeders no longer wanted these stallions, because the use of the trotters produced lighter horses. As a consequence, the breeding policies changed, and the cold-blooded trotters were no longer allowed to breed in the Døle. The effect of this decision was extreme, and within 5-10 years the level of inbreeding was higher than ever, with an average in the reference population of about 12% at the end of the 1990's. As an initiative today, a north-swedish breed (Nordsvensk brukshäst) is temporarily used in the Døle, but this is not a good long-term solution.

The Nordland/Lyngen has had a relatively high level of inbreeding for many years, without sudden changes in the past 40-50 years. The high level in this breed is no surprise, as one stallion born in 1935, at a time when ensuring the survival of the breed was the main priority, contributed 26% to the reference population (result not shown).

For both breeds it will be important to gain control over the selection with optimum contribution. This will minimize the average coancestry of parents and thus also the level of inbreeding of the next generation (Sonesson & Meuwissen, 2001). There are no recent reports of serious health damages in these two breeds, although there is no systematic recording of such data. For one thing, it would be important to record fertility data to survey possible reductions in fitness over time. A database is expected to be established in 2005 by the Norwegian Equine Centre, in which all matings and all animals born can be recorded.

The level of inbreeding in the reference populations was high in both breeds, with an average that is nearly equivalent to half-sib matings. Both breeds had low effective population sizes, compared with the recommended minimum size of approximately 100 (Klemetsdal, 1999). The complexity of calculating a reliable F is shown in the different periods when using regression, as the approximate values of ΔF and thus also N_e change considerable when including larger time periods. This paper therefore also considered use of a complementary approach by analysing the probabilities of gene origin.

When calculating the different probabilities of gene origin, the organisation of the data was an important challenge. The organisation we used when computing the effective number of founders, with each individual listed with all its respective ancestors in each generation, is necessary to get an overview and to get different parameters for pedigree completeness. However, Boichard *et al.* (1997)'s algorithm is simpler and should have preference in calculation of f_e, if the sole aim is to calculate this parameter. This algorithm is also a part of the algorithm described to calculate the effective number of ancestors. Since our starting point all the time was our defined reference population, it was a natural definition of generation t when calculating the effective number of founder genomes. To cover all the relevant elements in their relationship matrix, the dummy-individuals were created by the imaginary matings between all possible combinations in the reference population, which gave us the most exact calculation of the average coancestry.

The effective number of founders in the Døle was 48, which is only a small fraction of the actual number of founders in the pedigree. This shows the skewness in the contributions, and that only a few founders have contributed in some extent to our reference population. In the Nordland/Lyngen, which has another history of registration, the balance of the founder contributions is less skewed compared to the Døle, although yet imbalanced. When accounting for possible bottlenecks, the effective number of ancestors falls to approximately 10 individuals in both breeds. And finally, when the probability of gene loss by drift is considered, the smallest number is found; the effective number of founder genomes, which is just around 4-5 for both breeds. In all these measures, the Nordland/Lyngen has slightly lower values than the Døle.

It is shown that the use of inbreeding coefficients alone, as a tool to describe the genetic variation in a population, can be insufficient and misleading. The use of probabilities of gene origin is more robust, and allows us to account for different kinds of realities a population is exposed to through the generations. It is a complementary approach, and in our case the values calculated in the Døle and in the Nordland/Lyngen strongly indicate that the genetic variation could be reduced, and that the situation has become much more alarming than reported in Vangen (1983). As a consequence, the breeds should carefully plan future breeding, where the aim must be to recover the genetic variation. It is not recommended to carry out strong selection of any kind, as this will further worsen the problems of inbreeding and genetic drift. The focus should be on selection with optimum contribution (Sonesson & Meuwissen, 2001), which is an effective tool that can also prevent the need for introduction of unrelated genetic material from another breed, which is not considered as a good long-term solution when the aim is to conserve the original breeds. In this context, a simulation is planned to compare the actual breeding situation with a number of alternative strategies for genetic conservation.

References

Ballou, J.D. and R.C. Lacy, 1995. Identifying genetically important individuals for management of genetic variation in pedigreed populations. In: Ballou, J.D., Gilpin, M. and Foose, T.J. (eds.) Population management for survival and recovery, Columbia University Press, New York, pp. 76-111.

Boichard, D., L. Maignel and É. Verrier, 1997. The value of using probabilities of gene origin to measure genetic variability in a population. Genet. Sel. Evol. 29, 5-23.

Caballero, A. and M.A. Toro, 2000. Interrelations between effective population size and other pedigree tools for the management of conserved populations. Genet. Res. Camb. 75, 331-343.

Falconer, D.S. and T.F.C. Mackay, 1996. Introduction to quantitative genetics, 4th edn. Longman Group, Essex, England, 464 pp.

Fridrichsen, A., 1961. Utviklingen av kaldblodstraveravlen i Norge. In: P. Gjestvang, A. Fridrichsen and E.K. Aamot (Eds.). Boken om hesten. Vårt Forlag AS, Oslo, pp. 323-345. (In Norwegian).

Gaustad, M., 1951. Noen betraktninger om årets hingsteutstilling på Bjerke og om hesteavlen i sin alminnelighet. Våre Hester Sommernummer 1951, 6-7. (In Norwegian).

Gaustad, M., 1953. Statens utstilling for dølehingster. Dølehestavlen. In: S. Rohdin (Editor). Våre Hester Julenummer, 14-17. (In Norwegian).

Henderson, C.R., 1976. A simple method for computing the inverse of a numerator relationship matrix used in prediction of breeding values. Biometrics 32, 69-83.

Klemetsdal, G., 1999. Stochastic simulation of sire selection strategies in North-Swedish and Norwegian cold-blooded trotters. Livest. Prod. Sci. 57, 219-229.

Lacy, R.C., 1989. Analysis of founder representation in pedigrees: Founder equivalents and founder genome equivalents. Zoo Biol. 8, 111-123.

Lacy, R.C., 1995. Clarification of terms and their use in the management of captive populations. Zoo Biol. 14, 565-578.

MacCluer, J.W., J.L. VandeBerg, B. Read and O. Ryder, 1986. Pedigree analysis by computer simulation. Zoo Biol. 5, 147-160.

Quaas, R.L., 1976. Computing the diagonal elements and inverse of a large numerator relationship matrix. Biometrics 32, 949-953.
Rochambeau, H. de, L.F. de La Fuente, R. Rouvier and J. Ouhayoun, 1989. Sélection sur la vitesse de croissance post-sevrage chez le lapin. Genet. Sel. Evol. 21, 527-546.
Ruane, J., 2000. A framework for prioritizing domestic animal breeds for conservation purposes at the national level: a Norwegian case study. Conservation Biology 14, 1385-1393.
Sonesson, A. and T.H.E. Meuwissen, 2001. Minimization of rate of inbreeding for small populations with overlapping generations. Genet. Res., Camb. 77, 285-292.
Vangen, O., 1983. The use of relationship matrices to avoid inbreeding in small horse populations. Z. Tierzûchtg. Zûchtsbiol. 100, 48-54.
Zechner, P., J. Sölkner, T. Druml, R. Baumung, R. Achmann, I. Bodo, E. Marti, F. Habe and G. Brem, 2002. Analysis of diversity and population structure in the Lipizzan horse breed based on pedigrees information. Livest. Prod. Sci. 77, 137-146.

Bardigiano horse selection: a genetic global index for linear type traits

M. Fioretti[1], *A.L. Catalano*[2], *A. Rosati*[3] *and F. Martuzzi*[2]

[1]*AIA (Associazione Italiana Allevatori), Via G. Tomassetti 9, 00161 Rome, Italy*
[2]*Dip. Produzioni Animali, Università degli Studi, Via del Taglio 8, 43100 Parma, Italy*
[3]*EAAP (European Association for Animal Production), Via Nomentana 134, 00162 Rome, Italy*

Abstract

The selection of the Bardigiano Horse, an ancient work breed of the mountain areas in Parma and Piacenza Provinces (Northern Italy), is now oriented to produce horses for saddle service; at present, a genetic index for "height at withers" is used to obtain taller horses; in order to consider more traits, important for the Bardigiano Horse typicalness, a global genetic index (IGG) has been created, using traits from the linear morphological evaluation form. To obtain IGG, 18 different traits were genetically evaluated by BLUP –AM. The model accounted for the following effects: additive genetic, herd group evaluation by evaluation year, month of birth, age at evaluation in months and sex of evaluated animal. Heritability, genetic and environmental correlation for the morphological linear evaluation form traits and withers height were estimated. To take into account the different variability of studied traits, the genetic index of each trait was standardized. Finally, each standardized index was corrected for a specific weight in IGG composition and corrected indexes were added to obtain IGG. Genetic trend, calculated from year 1985 to year 2000 for males and females, was positive.

Keywords: Bardigiano, horse, genetic index, linear type traits

Introduction

Bardigiano horse is an ancient Italian breed, mainly reared in northern Italy, in the Appenine zone among Emilia-Romagna, Toscana and Liguria regions.

Bardigiano horses are bay and black in color, with withers height ranging from 135 to 145 centimeters and live weight of 450-550 kg. Animals have good temper, light head, small and neat ears, a thick mane crest and strong neck. Chest is deep and wide as withers. Back region is straight with medium length, rump is wide with correct slope, legs are short and muscled with pronounced joints, short cannon bone and hard hooves. A general body strength and ruggedness characterizes this breed.

The roots of this breed are deeply connected to the events in the origin area. This hilly zone was a transit from northern Italy to Rome and from Rome to Santiago de Compostela (via Francigena). In years 1250-1682 the zone was ruled by Landi family, defended by the castles of Bardi, Compiano and Borgo Val Taro; local horses were used for military purposes. Afterwards, horses were used mainly for farm uses. Therefore in this hilly area a "mountain" horse local population was living, turning to be more and more homogeneous. Only mares were of interest because mated to donkey stallions to produce mules, whose price was twice the price for a horse. Stallions were not reared. Even Italian Army used, from 1925 to 1945, Bardigiano mares for mule production (Bigliardi, 1988).

In 1930 this horse population was defined as "Bardigiano" horse, from Bardi, a town where the interest for this breed was great due to tradition, and where the highest number of animals was reared.

In the Seventies, in Parma and Piacenza, a census was made on Bardigiano population: in 1974, the population comprised 5 stallions and 94 mares. In 1977, Bardigiano Horse Studbook was instituted with several aims: to check birth events and ownership, to perform selection by evaluation of animals, fertility tests on stallions and planned matings, to organize meetings and in general to promote the diffusion and knowledge of the breed (Catalano, 1980).

From 1977 to 1993 Bardigiano was raised for meat production only. As a consequence of several factors, such its numerical decrease and the low revenues on horsemeat production, in 1993 it was decided to change selection goals in order to define new application fields for this breed. It was decided to raise Bardigiano mainly for saddle service and light draft, leaving meat production as a secondary purpose (Catalano & Martuzzi, 1994).

Bardigiano horses are perfectly adapted to different altitudes and climates. They have low feeding requirements, are resistant to drought periods, adapt themselves to climatic changes and stand each type of fodder and pasture. The housing system of the animals is free-range in the pastures from May to November and recovered in barns in wintertime only. Colts, born during spring months (from April to June), are sold during the autumn for meat production (with the only exception of future stallions) while fillies are raised to be mares.

In year 2001, 3400 Bardigiano horses were estimated to be in Italy, 2380 recorded in the Studbook (1522 mares, 105 stallions, and 769 young animals) reared in 666 herds. Table 1 shows the official statistics for number of animals and herds for Italy in years 1997-2001.

Table 1. Number of animals and herds in Italy in years 1997-2001 (source: Bardigiano Studbook).

Year	1997	1998	1999	2000	2001
Total estimated population	3500	3400	3400	3400	3400
Studbook population	2100	2060	2190	2370	2380
Live Studbook Mares	1214	1242	1376	1510	1522
Live Studbook Stallions	90	95	98	101	105
Studbook Herds	583	584	600	657	666

Table 2 shows Studbook statistics for number of animals and herds in Italy in year 2001 by regions, and for Germany, Hungary and Switzerland.

Selection aims to obtain animals suitable for saddle service and light draft purposes, increasing their withers height, body development and reproductive precocity, their fertility and length of productive life, preserving, at the same time, their natural body strength and ruggedness that allow the animals to live outside the barn, and to produce, at least, an appreciable amount of meat with low productive costs.

Table 2. Number of animals and herds in Italy in year 2001 by regions, and in Germany, Hungary and Switzerland. (source: Bardigiano Studbook)

Italian Region	N. herds	Mares	Stallion	Young	Total
Valle d' Aosta	1	1	=	=	1
Piemonte	20	29	2	15	46
Lombardia	29	48	5	47	100
Friuli Venezia Giulia	2	6	1	1	8
Veneto	1	2	=	3	5
Emilia Romagna	412	946	80	439	1465
Liguria	150	398	15	222	635
Toscana	47	85	2	26	113
Lazio	2	2	=	=	2
Abruzzo	1	3	=	=	3
Sicilia	1	2	=	=	2
Total	666	1522	105	769	2380
Country	**N. Herds**	**Mares**	**Stallion**	**Young**	**Total**
Hungary	1	2	=		2
Germany	20	28	2	5	35
Switzerland	1	=	2	=	2

Genetic evaluation is based on a BLUP-Animal Model procedure (Samorè & Rosati, 1995), like in other horse Italian breeds: *e.g.* Haflinger, Italian Heavy Draught Horse (Mantovani *et al.*, 2004; Pagnacco & Samorè, 2003). Since one of the most important selection aspect was to obtain animals suitable for riding, withers height (expressed in cm) together with other longitudinal measurements were the only traits of interest for selection and, due to a high positive correlation among them, animals were genetically evaluated and selected for withers height. Heritability for withers height was 0.64, meaning that the trait was influenced just a little by environmental effects and much more by genetic effects so that response to selection could be fast for both sexes.

In the Haflinger breed as well selection was focused since 1990 on the production of taller horses for country riding. Heritability for withers height in that breed is 0.75 (Pagnacco & Samorè, 2003).

Withers height index (IGA) was calculated from a single trait BLUP – AM evaluation for withers height trait. The model was:

$$Y_{ijklm} = A_i + HY_j + M_k + Sex_l + b_1*Age_m + b_1*Age^2_m + b_1*Age^3_m + e_{ijklm}$$

Where:

Y_{ijklm}	= withers height on the ith horse;
A_i	= animal additive genetic effect for the ith horse;
HY_j	= fixed effect of the jth "herd group evaluation by evaluation year";
M_k	= fixed effect of horse's k^{th}month of birth class (3 classes);
Sex_l	= fixed effect of horse l^{th} sex;
Age_m	= horse age at evaluation, expressed in months;
b_1, b_2, b_3	= linear, quadratic and cubic regression coefficients for age in months;
e_{ijklm}	= error.

IGA derived from withers height EBVs corrected for a genetic base consisting in average EBV value for mares born in 1995. Italian Breeders Association (A.I.A.) Research Office is in charge of IGA calculation yearly.

Development of the Genetic Global Index (IGG)

Both Studbook and A.I.A. Research Office realised that a selection involving also other body conformation traits could be a great step ahead for a more complete improvement of this breed for the aimed selection goals. For this reason AIA Research Office studied and developed a new selection index, called *Genetic Global Index (IGG)* adding to withers height other traits recorded in the morphologic linear evaluation by Studbook. (Score for linear evaluation for each trait could range from 1 to 10).

The 18 considered traits are shown in Table 3. These traits differ from those taken in account for the Haflinger horse, breed with similar selection objective, where 26 traits are considered: also gaits and temperament are taken in account, showing a higher emphasis toward a sport horse in this breed, and 3 are about coat colour (Samoré *et al.*, 1997).

Table 3. Evaluated traits for IGG.

Trait
Withers Height
Head volume
Head profile
Head expression
Neck length
Neck – trunk connection
Shoulder length
Shoulder slope
Thorax and breast, front view
Back –loin line, withers
Back –loin line, length
Back –loin line, direction
Rump length
Rump slope
Rump width
Legs quality
Front legs, stance
Rear legs, behind view

In the Italian Heavy Draught Horse instead the selection purposes are to produce a horse with big muscular masses for meat production, and an energetic stride for harness competitions. Therefore 2 trait are considered, called "fleshiness" and "blood".

Morphological trait classes were, where necessary, expressed as deviations from the scoring class considered to be optimal, that is the "ideal value" representing the correct value that an ideal Bardigiano horse should have for that particular trait.

A single trait BLUP – AM was used to predict EBVs for each of 18 traits. For withers height, EBVs were already calculated for IGA (withers height index).

Table 4. Heritabilities for traits used in IGG composition.

Trait	Heritability
Withers Height	0.64
Head volume	0.47
Head profile	0.33
Head expression	0.39
Neck length	0.04
Neck – trunk connection	0.22
Shoulder length	0.08
Shoulder slope	0.03
Thorax and breast, front view	0.39
Back –loin line, withers	0.04
Back –loin line, length	0.08
Back –loin line, direction	0.17
Rump length	0.17
Rump slope	0.22
Rump width	0.25
Legs quality	0.11
Front legs, stance	0.09
Rear legs, behind view	0.09

Heritabilities for each trait (Fioretti & Rosati, unpublished work) are reported in Table 4. EBVs were predicted using the following mixed model (single trait BLUP – AM):

$$Y_{ijklm} = A_i + HY_j + M_k + Sex_l + b_1 * Age_m + b_1 * Age^2_m + b_1 * Age^3_m + e_{ijklm}$$

Where:

Y_{ijklm} = trait of the the ith horse;
A_i = animal additive genetic effect for the ith horse;
HY_j = fixed effect of the jth "herd group evaluation by evaluation year";
M_k = fixed effect of horse's kth month of birth class (3 classes);
Sex_l = fixed effect of horse lth sex;
Age_m = horse age at evaluation, expressed in months;
b_1, b_2, b_3 = linear, quadratic and cubic regression coefficients for age in months;
e_{ijklm} = error.

Basically, the model was the same used for IGA. Only HY groups of at least two records were used. Herd groups were created considering homogeneous management effects tied to geographical zones. For each animal, EBVs for all the considered traits were predicted, then they were standardized, in order to make EBVs from different traits comparable among themselves. Bardigiano Studbook Technical Committee provided "weights" for each trait in order to compute an aggregate genetic index. Weights were expressed as multiplicative coefficients expressing the relative importance of a trait in the constitution of the "ideal" Bardigiano horse. Weights are reported in Table 5.

The Global Genetic Index (IGG) was calculated by multiplying, for each trait, its standardized EBVs by its "weight". Results for each trait were then added together, yielding the Global Genetic Index. Genetic base was average IGG for females born in 1995. Italian Breeders Association (A.I.A.) Research Office is in charge of IGG calculation yearly.

Table 5. Trait weights in IGG calculation.

Trait	Weight
Withers Height	0.30
Head volume	0.03
Head profile	0.03
Head expression	0.04
Neck length	0.03
Neck – trunk connection	0.02
Shoulder length	0.03
Shoulder slope	0.02
Thorax and breast, front view	0.05
Back –loin line, withers	0.04
Back –loin line, length	0.03
Back –loin line, direction	0.03
Rump length	0.06
Rump slope	0.04
Rump width	0.05
Legs quality	0.05
Front legs, stance	0.05
Rear legs, behind view	0.05

Use of Genetic Global Index

From year 2001, the two genetic indexes for Bardigiano, IGA and IGG, are used together as selection tools. Stallions are used for reproduction if their IGA are greater or equal +1 cm and their IGG is positive and their global score is equal or greater than 83 points; mares are selected if they have at least both parents in Studbook, the best rank for IGA in their herd's province, a positive IGG and global score equal or greater than 80.

Selection results

Genetic trend for IGA and IGG are reported in Figure 1 and Figure 2. The high trend increase in population obtained from 1993 to 2001 is mainly due to accurate selection activity of Studbook and to the high withers height heritability value. Trend increasing is more evident and has fewer variations in female population due to higher number of females. Male populations, with a low animal number, show a high variation in IGA and IGG per birth year, but an evident increasing trend has been obtained from 1994 to 2001. Both IGA and IGG show the same trend, since withers height influence IGG for 30%.

Additional selective tools: inbreeding monitoring

Bardigiano breed is a small population and considering that each year only few males are used as stallions, it becomes extremely important to check inbreeding level, avoiding its increase among population. A.I.A. Research Office checks yearly inbreeding among all population (dead and alive animals) and among living animals only.

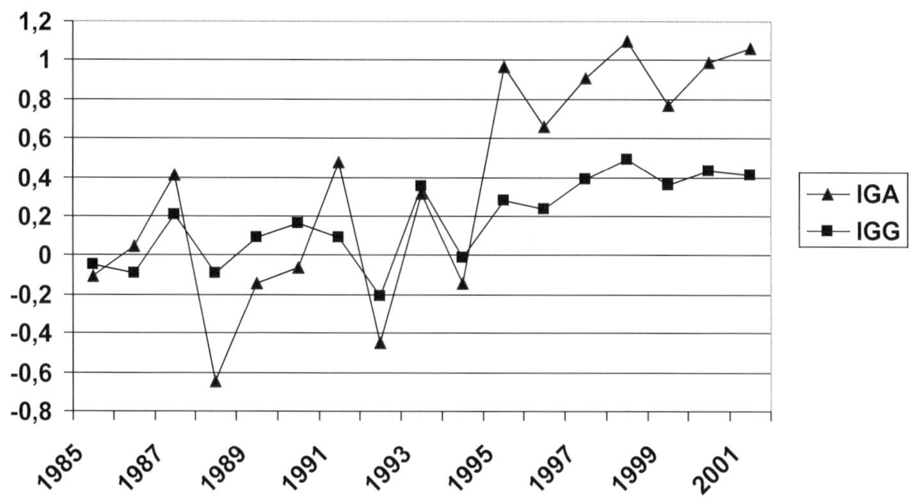

Figure 1. Genetic trend for IGA and IGG, Bardigiano males.

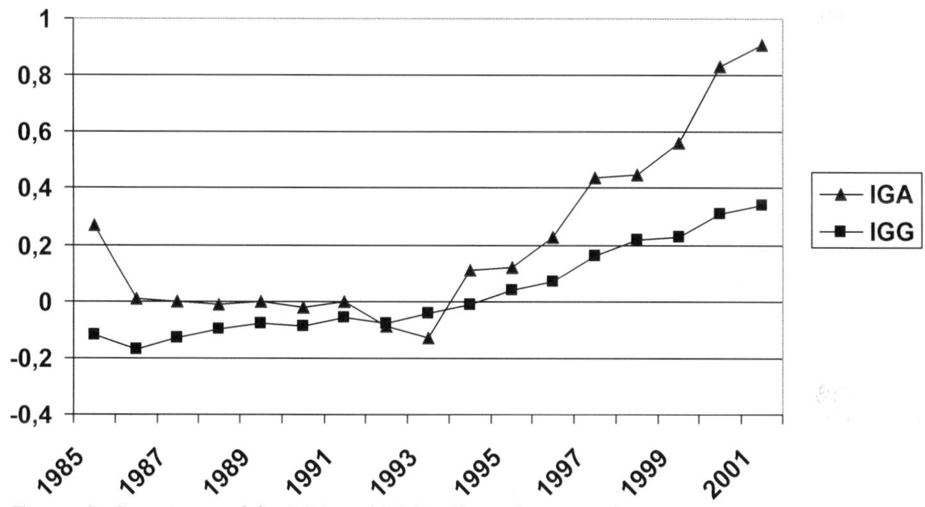

Figure 2. Genetic trend for IGA and IGG, all Bardigiano subjects.

Moreover, a routine procedure has been developed in order to simulate all possible matings for all living animals in the population; progeny inbreeding from each of these possible matings is computed. In this way, Bardigiano Studbook is able to avoid mating between animals that will have inbred progeny. Particularly farmers are informed about which stallion, whenever mated to farm mares, will produce an offspring with inbreeding greater than 5%.

The variability of the breed was investigated by gene frequencies for several loci in a survey carried out in 1980 about haematic genetic markers, and a good genetic variability was demonstrated (Cristofalo *et al.*, 1989). Since then some studies about molecular genetics in other Italian horse breeds except the Bardigiano breed have been carried out considering mainly mitochondrial DNA (Cozzi *et al.*, 2003; Cozzi *et al.*, 2004).

Conclusions

The introduction of Genetic Global Index in Bardigiano horse selection allows to take into account not only horse's height, but also to improve at the same time desired conformation for peculiar morphological traits.

Withers height still has a high influence in IGG composition (30%). With the introduction of Global Genetic Index (IGG) besides Withers Height Index (IGA), and their contemporary use in selection, it will be possible to go on selecting animals for higher withers height improving, at the same time, general conformation of the breed to desirable standards.

Genetic trends for both IGG and IGA show an increasing trend, more marked in females. Application of this new selection index could help Bardigiano breeders to obtain animals suitable for tourism purposes, maintaining a link between the breed and its own environment, and to increase breed popularity as well as total number of Bardigiano horses.

It is important anyway to check the response to selection, adjusting constantly the weight of the different selected traits in order to satisfy the priorities of the breeders and considering the evolution of morphology and performance shaped by selection.

Acknowledgement

The authors wish to thank for his remarkable cooperation in this study Gianpaolo Pagani (Associazione Nazionale Allevatori Cavallo di Razza Bardigiana)

References

Bigliardi, E., 1988. Cavallo e Territorio. Il Bardigiano nelle valli Taro e Ceno. Ed. Az. Comunale Diritto allo Studio – Parma

Catalano, A.L., 1980. Bardigiano horse. Distintive feature of mares registered on stud book. La Clinica Veterinaria, 103, 9-10.

Catalano, A.L. and F. Martuzzi, 1994. Diffusione, variabilità morfologica ed evoluzione della razza cavallina Bardigiana. Annali Fac. Medicina Veterinaria, Università di Parma, Vol. XIV.

Cozzi, M.C., M.G. Strillacci, P. Valiati, B. Bighignoli, M. Cancedda and M. Zanotti, 2003. Study of mitochondrial D-loop DNA sequence variation in some Italian horse breeds. Proc. 5th Meeting "New findings in equine practice", 33-39.

Cozzi, M.C., M.G. Strillacci, P. Valiati, B. Bighignoli, M. Cancedda and M. Zanotti, 2004. Mitochondrial D-loop sequence variation among Italian horse breeds. Genet. Sel. Evol., 36, 663-672.

Cristofalo, C., M.C. Cozzi, A. Mezzelani and A.L. Catalano, 1989. Analysis of the Bardigiano Horse breed by haematic genetic markers. Proceedings 9th Meeting of the Italian Association of Equine Practitioners, 85-88.

Mantovani, R., G. Pigozzi, I. Cerchiaro and L. Bailoni, 2004. Results of genetic improvement in the Italian Heavy Draught Horse. Proc. 6th Meeting "New findings in equine practice", 43-49.

Pagnacco, G. and A.B. Samoré, 2003. Recent History and selection perspective in Italian Haflinger Horse. Proc. 5th Meeting "New findings in equine practice", 9-23.

Samoré, A.B., G. Pagnacco and F. Miglior, 1997. Genetic parameters and breeding values for linear type traits in the Haflinger horse. Livest. Prod. Sci., 52, 105-111.

Samoré, A.B. and A. Rosati, 1995. Animal Model estimation of breeding values for Bardigiano horse breed. Book of Abstract of the 46th Annual Meeting of the E.A.A.P., Prague, 1995.

The Italian Heavy Draught Horse breed: origin, breeding program, efficiency of the selection scheme and inbreeding

R. Mantovani[1], G. Pigozzi[2] and G. Bittante[1]

[1]*Department of Animal Science, University of Padova. Agripolis, Viale dell'Università 16, 35020 Legnaro (PD), Italy*
[2]*Italian Heavy Draught Horse Breeders Association, Via del Belgio 10, 37135 Verona, Italy*

Abstract

At present Italian Heavy Draught Horse (IHDH) is bred not only for rapid draught but mainly for meat production. The current IHDH population consists of about 6700 animals (3300 mares, 3000 foals of 6-30 months of age and 400 stallions) registered in the studbook. The IHDH usually has a chestnut coat with fair hair and it can reach an adult body weight of about 900 kg in the stallion. It is recognized to belong to the French Heavy subgroup breeds, due to the past and present use of French Breton stallions on IHDH mares. In the mare the mean productive life is about 5.8 years with a mean production of 4.5 foals; the foals show a mean growth rate of 1 kg/d, a slaughter weight that reach about 430 kg and a cold dressing percentage of 61%. The selection scheme is based on a linear type evaluation of the 2-7 month aged foals, scoring 11 traits belonging to 3 main groups (general aspect, trunk and legs). Results obtained with the selection programme employed for the IHDH indicate that the generation interval is progressively shortening both in the stallions and in the mares (6.1 and 6.5 years, respectively), but a further reduction could be expected for the stallions as soon as the incidence of the artificial insemination will be increased in the future. The genetic trend for "fleshiness" score has increased rapidly in the last decade of selection (+2.6% and +3.9% of the phenotypic mean for mares and stallions, respectively), although other traits as "blood" have increased slowly, particularly for the stallions rather than for the mares (+0.5% vs. +1.8% of the phenotypic mean, respectively). Despite the reduced population size, the annual increase in inbreeding coefficient was found to be very low (+0.07%/year) for the IHDH population.

Keywords: Italian Heavy Draught Horse, origin, breeding program, selection efficiency, inbreeding

Introduction

In recent years the horse production in Italy has rapidly increased in number due to a growing interest for horse-racing and riding. Indeed, almost all Italian breed have seen an increased number of registered animals in their studbook. This phenomenon has interested also the Italian Heavy Draught Horse (IHDH), although this breed is mainly selected today for meat production than for rapid draught as in the past. However, an increased number of farms have introduced this breed beside the cattle and the breeding area of IHDH has been widespread within the country territory.

The aim of this paper is to describe the IHDH population, its relationship with other breeds and to point out the selection scheme adopted for this breed. Moreover, this paper is aimed to analyze the selection efficiency in terms of generation interval and genetic trend obtained during almost 10 years of selection activity and, due to the reduced population size, the inbreeding rate through generation.

The Italian Heavy Draught Horse: story and characteristics

The origin of the Italian Heavy Draught Horse (IHDH) is related to the need of developing a strain of heavy horse in Italy to be used in rapid draught for both agriculture and field artillery. This project was first supported by military programs that started just after the Kingdom of Italy was established in 1861, and was at first based on crosses between European heavy stallions (mainly from Norfolk-Breton crosses better known as "Posthorse" or "Postier Breton") and heavy mares locate in studs widespread mainly in the North-east of Italy. However, an official mating registration program of foals obtained from selected mares started only in 1927. Newborn females and males from the first registered generation were then used to build up new Italian families of horses beside the Breton derived animals. During the 30's the objective of a more homogeneous female base was followed together with the development of functional and morphological evaluation of stallions aged 3 and 4 years. This process was partially interrupted by the 2nd world war, but during the 50's the breeding area of IHDH was extended to many studs in the centre and in the south of Italy, that introduced IHDH stallions for to get heavier horses to be used in agriculture. To this increase in weight and size have greatly contributed the Breton stallions, which over years have been used on IHDH breed. Indeed, the EAAP-animal genetic data bank (www.tiho-hannover.de/einricht/zucht/eaap/index.htm, 2005) classify the IHDH within the subgroup of French heavy horses together with French Breton, Boulonnais, Poitou and Percheron, and stallions from the French Breton population are still allowed to be used on IHDH mares. However, within the main Italian horse breed, the IHDH shows almost unique characteristics, as recently demonstrated using microsatellite markers by Bruzzone *et al.* (2003). This could be probably related also to the uniqueness of this heavy breed in the country territory, which is not common in other EU country, where a greater number of draught breed are available, although well differentiated from the genetic point of view (Aberle *et al.*, 2004). On the other hand, a more accurate analysis of the relationship among the IHDH and other EU heavy draught breeds, has recently done for the Lipizzan horse (Achmann *et al.*, 2004), seem nowadays strictly necessary. The establishment of the IHDH studbook dated back to 1960, but after this, during the two subsequent decades a decline of interest for the IHDH in the big farms located in the north-east of Italy due to the mechanization of agriculture was observed. However, during the '70s and '80s, the interest for the IHDH moved from the use for "traction" to the meat production in both the small northern farms and in the biggest farms located in the centre and in the south of Italy. The new selection purpose and the management of the studbook by the National Breeders Association (established in 1968 from a previous Breeders Association founded in Verona in 1946), has led during the 80's to an extension of the selection base up to the present population size, that account for about 6700 registered animals (3300 mares and 400 stallions) in 980 registered herds widespread in almost all the country. The IHDH is nowadays a bulky animal with a mature body weight that can reach 900 kg in the stallions. The minimum height at withers for animals of 30 months of age is 146 cm for the females and 150 cm for the stallions, but a preferred height of 155-160 for males and 150-158 for mares is suggested. The coat is usually chestnut with fair hair (sometimes white), although some animals are red roan or bay (about 20% of incidence). Table 1 shows the main characteristics of the Italian Heavy Draught Horse.

Table 1. Main characteristics of IHDH animals.

Mares:		
- age at 1st foaling	yrs.	3.5
- age at culling	yrs.	9.3
- productive life (PL)	yrs.	5.8
- conceptions during PL	no.	4.7
- foals during PL	no.	4.5
- mean foals/PL		0.78
- mean foaling rate		0.82
Foals:		
- slaughter weight	kg	431
- cold dressing percentage	%	61

Lifetime in the registered IHDH mares is 9.3 years, although with a high variability, since 32% of mares have shown a lifespan higher than 10 years of age. Fertility data in the IHDH mares (studbook reproductive statistics, 2004; unpublished) appear to be very high, with a mean foaling rate of 82% and a mean number of 4.5 foals produced during the 5.8 years of productive life. These results and, particularly, the foaling rate, are higher than data reviewed by Gordon (1997) for thoroughbred, and indicate a good level of fertility for a breed that has no relationship with sport or related activities. Together with the good fertility and the reasonable lifespan, the IHDH shows good meat production ability. Indeed, data recorded by the IHDH breeder association (studbook, 2004; unpublished) indicate a dressing percentage of 61% in foals aged about 15 months and slaughtered at about 430 kg after weaning at pasture and subsequent fattening in stable. Therefore, under these circumstances the IHDH foals exhibit a growth rate of about 1.0 kg/d, which is in agreement with values reported by Trillaud-Geyl *et al.* (1984), for the French yearlings belonging to heavy breeds and fattened under similar circumstances. IHDH selection has a dual purpose, although the main selection goal is meat production and, only in the recent years, there has been an increasing interest for the rapid draught in the horse team races and in the use of horses for the agricultural work in the organic farming systems or in the woods.

The selection scheme adopted for the Italian Heavy Draught Horse

The selection scheme set up for the IHDH is based on the genetic evaluation for linear type traits recorded on foals since 1993. The linear type evaluation involves the scoring of 11 traits using a 5 point scale (based on a biological scale), by a group of classifiers that evaluate yearly foals aged between 2 and 7 months. These traits belong to 3 main groups: 1) general aspect (head size and expression and neck direction - HSD, blood - BL, frame size, fleshiness – FL, and bone incidence), 2) trunk (thorax depth, fore – FD and rear diameters -RD, length and direction of upper line), 3) leg traits (side view of rear legs). Together with the evaluation of the foals, classifiers also provide a linear type evaluation (8 traits only) and a condition score on 3 point scale (lean, medium and fat) for the mares. Using a multivariate animal model, heritability and genetic correlation among traits have been computed and routinely breeding values are estimated (setting the mean EBV at 100 and the standard deviation at 10). The model for the genetic evaluation accounts for the fixed effects of classifier, sex and age of the foal at score (in classes of 1 month) and age of the mare at score (in classes of 1 year). The effects herd-year of evaluation and animal are also included in the model but as random effects. About the herd-year effect, it has to be pointed out that due to the small size of many herds and to the reduced incidence of the AI (i.e. the use of a single stallion in a group of mares), only a small amount of herd-year classes are actual farms within a given year of evaluation. Grouping of farms with foals from a single stallion is based as for Italian Haflinger on geographical region and management (Samorè *et al.*, 1997), but also considering different farm's production objective (meat or draught), foal prophylaxis and mean condition score of the mares. Heritability used for estimating breeding values ranges from 8 to 23%, with FL that exhibits the highest value. Selection is made on the basis of a Total Selection Index (TSI) that accounts for HSD (25%), BL (15%), FL (25%), FD (15%) and RD (20%), whose are the most important traits for the selection goal defined by the National Breeders Association. Thus, if the linear type trait classification allows getting both field performance (for foals) and progeny (for stallions and mares) tests, the third moment of the selection scheme is the admission of the animals to the studbook. Criteria for admission are supervised by the National Breeders Association through its technical committee and represent the way to control the genetic improvement process for the breed. Particularly, the access to the studbook is allowed for: 1) male foals with at least 3 generations of known ancestors, a minimum pedigree index for TSI of 100 and a minimum final morphological score of "good"; 2) female foals with a minimum final morphological score of "fair"; 3) stallions previously registered in the studbook as foals and with a breeding value for TSI of at least 100 for animals aged ≥3 years and a minimum TSI of 110 for animal younger stallion (i.e., aged 2 years). Due to the opening of the studbook to the French Breton population, registered Breton stallions and mares with at least 3 generations of known ancestors and a minimum final score of "very good" are allowed to be registered in the IHDH studbook.

Selection efficiency and inbreeding rate

Materials and methods

Data used in the study were:

- a pedigree of 38128 animals registered in the studbook in order to calculate the generation intervals for the sires of the sires and the dams of the dams;
- the genetic indexes for the linear type traits calculated by a BLUP animal model procedure (2054 mares and 109 stallions that had a progeny and were born after 1988) to estimate the genetic trend for BL and FL through a linear regression method;
- the estimation of the inbreeding from a database accounting for 21368 registered females (129 of which from the French Breton studbook) and 16760 males (145 French Bretons); inbreeding was obtained through the algorithm of VanRaden (1992) that computes the individual inbreeding coefficient adjusting for the missing pedigree information and the base population was set in 1970.

Simple descriptive statistics were obtained in analyzing the efficiency of the selection scheme and trends in inbreeding, while REGR procedure (SAS, 1990) was used to calculate the relationship between the inbreeding and the length of the productive life or the number of abortions/year of productive life.

Results and discussion

The actual generation interval for stallions (Table 2), calculated as age of a sire of sire at the birth of his first sons subsequently become a stallion, shows a mean value of 6.5 years, that could be considered a conventional value for a mammalian population where the reproductive career starts at about 3 years of age, and is characterized by a reduced reproductive efficiency, due to 11 months of gestation and to a low foaling rate (≤1/year). Moreover, this generation interval is close to that suggested as optimal for the male cattle undergone to a progeny test for the genetic evaluation (Van Vleck, 1979). Furthermore, the mean generation interval has shown a progressive reduction for each five year period considered, indicating a tendency to a general reduction in the age of the stallions used to get new stallions; indeed, both the standard deviation and the maximum age observed for a sire of sire have been both reduced during the years. Looking at the same kind of data obtained by tracing back the generations of the mares registered in the studbook, a trend similar to stallions has been observed in the female population, although some differences have to be remarked. Indeed, mares have shown a general mean value for generation interval a little lower than stallions (6.1 vs. 6.5 years, respectively), and have shown a marked decrease in this parameter only in the last five year period (Figure 1). All together, the generation intervals in both the pathways of the selection process indicate a general good agreement of farmers to the selection programme, particularly since the 90's, when an official programme was set up. On the other hand, it has to be pointed out that the shortening of the generation interval in both the selection pathways could not be expected to change rapidly in this species due to the limited use of the reproduction biotechnology, i.e. mares are not responsive to superovulation and stallions have a limited use in artificial insemination and only about 10% of foals born/year is obtained with this reproduction method. The actual genetic trend observed for the linear trait of BL has reached the value of 0.06 points per year for mares (Figure 2), which represents an increase of the 1.8% of the phenotypic mean. However, the trend for the same trait in the stallions has been quite lower, with an annual increase of 0.02 points (Figure 2), that corresponds to a 0.5% increase on the phenotypic mean, only. Similarly, the genetic trend for FL has shown a different genetic gain between mare and stallion, although in this case the mares have shown a lower annual increase in the genetic mean of the trait than the stallions (0.09 vs. 0.13 points/year, respectively; Figure 3).

Table 2. Descriptive statistics for generation interval in stallions.

Birth year period	Sire of sires	Sons/Stallion	Mean	s.d.	Min.	Max.
1975-1979	25	3.0	8.0	3.3	4.0	17.2
1980-1984	47	3.8	6.9	2.6	3.9	13.2
1985-1989	32	2.8	5.8	1.9	3.1	10.9
1990-1994	21	1.6	4.6	1.1	2.9	7.1
Overall	125	3.0	6.5	2.6	2.9	17.2

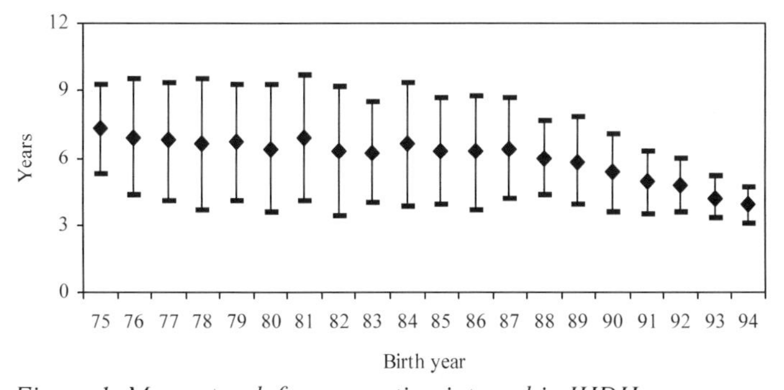

Figure 1. Means ± s.d. for generation interval in IHDH mares.

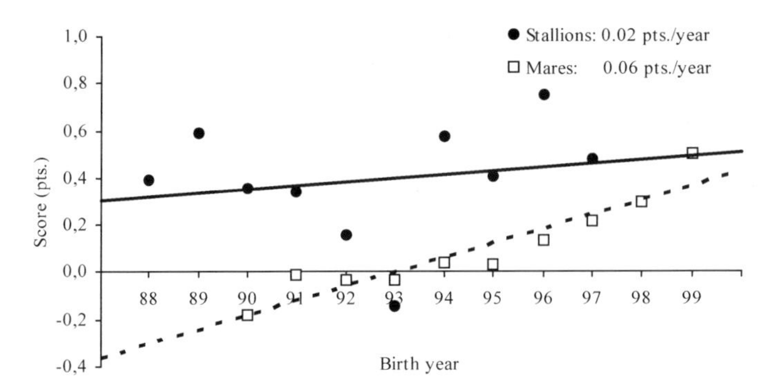

Figure 2. Genetic trend for linear score of the Blood trait.

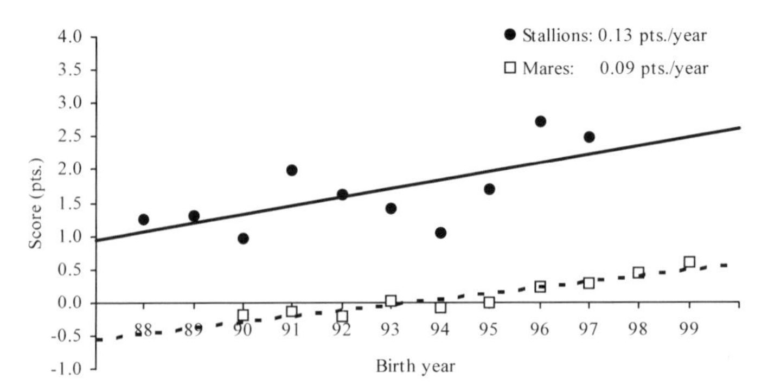

Figure 3. Genetic trend for linear score of Fleshiness trait.

However, the genetic gain for FL score has reached in both sexes a remarkable value, i.e. an increase of 2.6% and 3.9% of the phenotypic mean for mares and for the stallions, respectively. This result is probably due to the selection process applied in a population not previously selected on the basis of genetic indexes, and to the eminent interest addressed by farmers to this trait, particularly on the stallions, that have not been selected for BL if compare to the mare. Relatively to the 1970 population the Inbreeding coefficient (IC) ranged from 0.7 to 40.0%. The inbreeding level within the period of study was upwards, although the annual increase in the IC was generally lower than that suggested in literature (Falconer, 1989): +0.07%/year (Figure 4) and with only 1.6% of still alive animals (n=4900) that had an IC higher than 12.5%. The trends in the level of inbreeding showed a cyclic pattern over years, due to use of stallions imported from the French Breton population (FB; 87 animals from 1970). Indeed, stallions obtained by mating IHDH mares with FB stallions in the last decade showed a lower mean IC than those obtained within the IHDH population (2.90 vs. 4.35%), although the Breton animals from the French studbook are more related within group than the IHDH population. Indeed, the present still alive population indicates a higher percentage of animals with IC>12.5% within the animals of FB origin than within the IHDH population (9.4% vs. 1.5%). The coefficient obtained by regressing inbreeding with the length of productive life was not significant although it revealed an interesting negative relationship between inbreeding and length of life (Table 3). Probably due to the high variability observed for fertility parameter (such as for the lifetime) also the regression between inbreeding and foals/year or un-foaled/year was not significant (Table 3). The monitoring of inbreeding is of high interest in a small population since performance, health, fertility and survival are negatively affected by accumulation of inbreeding (Weigel, 2001). Moreover, in horses, racing performance (Klemetsdal, 1998), carpal joint arthritis (Dolvik and Klemetsdal, 1994) and retained placenta (Servinga *et al.*, 2004) have been demonstrated to be negatively correlated with inbreeding rate. Reviewing the inbreeding control in selection programs, Weigel (2001) indicated selection intensity as the main factor than can affect inbreeding, rather than population size. However, in small populations heritability of selected traits is generally lower (Meuwissen, 1997) and lower h^2 can lead to a more rapid accumulation of inbreeding (Strandén *et al.*, 1991). Despite the reduced population size and the possible rapid inbreeding accumulation, the trend of inbreeding detected for the IHDH population resulted very low and similar to that obtained by Moureaux *et al.* (1996) on Arab horses born in France and that estimated in Italy for Italian Haflinger horse (Gandini *et al.*, 1992).

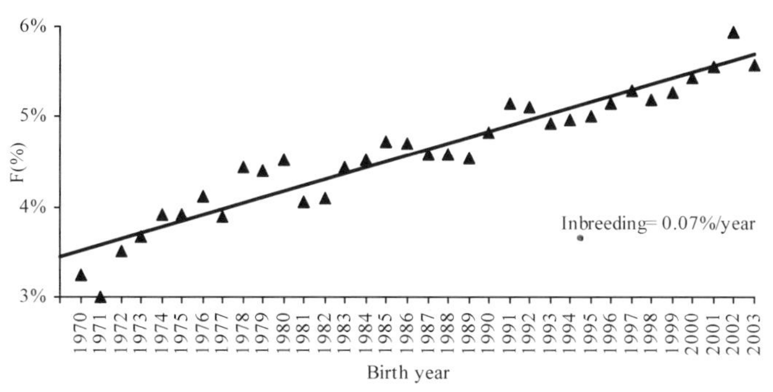

Figure 4. Trend for inbreeding in IHDH population.

Table 3. Relationship between inbreeding and lifetime or fertility parameters.

Variable	Regression coefficient	P
Length of life (months)	-2.96	n.s.
Foals/year of life (no.)	-0.11	n.s.
Un-foaled/year of life (no.)	0.05	n.s.

Conclusions

Although a selection process based on modern tools has started only recently, both the shortening of the generation interval toward normal values for a mammalian population and the genetic gain observed, particularly for the FL type trait, indicate that good results have been obtained in the genetic improvement programme of the IHDH. To this regard, a further reduction in the generation interval for the stallions, allowed by the increasing use of the AI, could be beneficial for the selection programme. Moreover the mean inbreeding rate observed over the years for the IHDH population resulted to be very low and of no great concern despite the small population size (i.e. about 3300 registered mares and 400 stallions). This is the result of the opening of the IHDH studbook both to the mares with an unknown pedigree but with a minimum morphological score and to the stallions from the French Breton population (87 animals imported from 1970 up to today). However a constant control of the inbreeding level appears to be necessary to optimise the selection scheme (Sonesson and Meuwissen, 2001). Finally, no significant relationships were found between inbreeding and lifetime or fertility traits.

References

Aberle, K.S., H. Hamann, C. Drögemüller and O. Distl, 2004. Genetic diversity in German draught horse breeds compared with a group of primitive, riding and wild horses by means of microsatellite DNA markers. Animal Genetics, 35, 270-277.

Achmann, R., I. Curik, P. Dovc, T. Kavar, I. Bodo, F. Habe, E. Marti, J. Sölkner and G. Brem, 2004. Microsatellite diversity, population subdivision and gene flow in the Lipizzan horse. Animal Genetics, 35, 285-292.

Bruzzone, A., D. Iamartino, M. Blasi and F. Pilla, 2003. The Pentro horse: genetic characterization by microsatellite markers. Ital. J. Anim. Sci., 2, 223-230.

Dolvik, N.I. and G. Klemetsdal, 1994. Arthritis in the carpal joints of Norvegian trotter-heritability, effects of inbreeding and conformation. Livest. Prod. Sci. 39, 283-290.

Falconer, D.S., 1989. Introduction to quantitative genetics. 3rd ed. Longman scientific & technical, Essex, England.

Gandini, G.C., A. Bagnato, F. Miglior and G. Pagnacco, 1992. Inbreeding in the Italian Haflinger horse. J. Anim. Breed. Genet., 109, 433-443.

Gordon, I., 1997. *Controlled reproduction in horses, deer and camelids*. CAB International, Wallingford, Oxon, UK, 1997.

Klemetsdal, G., 1998. The effect of inbreeding on racing performance in Norvegian cold-blooded trotters. Gen. Selec. Evol. 30, 351-366.

Meuwissen, T.H.E., 1997. Selection Scheme for small population.. 48th Annual Meeting of EAAP, Vienna, 25-28 August 1997.

Moureaux, S., E. Verrier, A. Ricard and J.C. Meriaux, 1995. Genetic variability within French race and riding horse breeds from genealogical data and blood marker polymorphisms. Gen. Selec. Evol. 28, 83-102.

Samorè, A.B., G. Pagnacco and F. Miglior, 1997. Genetic parameters and breeding values for linear type traits in the Haflinger horse. Livest. Prod. Sci., 52: 105-111.

SAS, 1990. SAS Procedure Guide. Ver. 6. 3rd Edition. SAS Institute Inc., Cary. NC, USA.

Servinga, M., T. Vrijenhoek, J.W. Hesselink, H.W. Barkema and A.F. Groen, 2004. Effect of inbreeding on the incidence of retained placenta in Friesian horses. J. Anim. Sci., 82, 982-986.

Sonesson, A.K. and T.H.E. Meuwissen, 2001. Minimum rate of inbreeding for small population with overlapping generations. Genetical Research, 77, 285-292.

Strandén I., A. Mäki-Tanila and E.A. Mäntysaari, 1991. Genetic progress and rate of inbreeding in a closed adult MOET nucleus under different mating strategies and heritabilities. J. Anim. Breed. Genet., 108, 401-411.

Trillaud-Geyl, C., M. Jussiaux, J. Agabriel and W. Martin-Rosset, 1984. Méthodes de production et d'alimentation à l'auge du poulain en croissance et à l'engrais. In: R. Jarrige, W. Martin-Rosset Ed., Le Cheval. Reproduction, sélection, alimentation, exploitation. INRA, Paris, 1984.

Van Vleck, D.L., 1979. *Notes on the theory and application of selection principles for the genetic improvement of animals*. Cornell Univ., Ithaca, NY.

VanRaden, P.M., 1992. Accounting for inbreeding and crossbreeding in genetic evaluation of large population. J. Dairy Sci. 75, 3136-3144.

Weigel, K.A., 2001. Controlling inbreeding in modern breeding programs. J. Dairy Sci. 84 (E. Suppl.), E177-E184.

Genetic characterization of Pentro young horses by microsatellite markers

D. Iamartino, M. Fidotti, N. Miraglia and F. Pilla

Molise University, Departement of Animals, Vegetables and Environmental Sciences, Via De Sanctis, 86100 Campobasso, Italy

Abstract

The Pentro horse population is an autochthonous breed from breeding area characterized by climatic and geographic peculiarity and today it counts about 400 heads. Because of its peculiar adaptive ability, the "Pentro Horse" must be considered a genetic resource which needs to be preserved. Moreover, the horse pasture is very important for the ecological equilibrium of the area. The genetic structure of Pentro population was studied by means of microsatellite markers (Bruzzone *et al.*, 2003) with the aim of the analysis of its biodiversity and relationship versus other horse breeds. The data introduced in this work regard the genetic and morphological assessment of Pentro young horses assigned to the reproduction demonstrating again the uniqueness and the identity of the Pentro group. A total of twelve microsatellite loci were used to score 23 Pentro young horses and then the obtained data were used to compare the genetic structure of the Pentro horse to other six Italian horse breeds (Maremmano, Murgese, TPR, Halflinger, Trottatore and Bardigiano). The genetic distance among individuals was calculated as the proportion of shared alleles, (Dps=1-Ps) according to Bowcock *et al.* (1994) using the Microsat software (Minch *et al.*, 1995). The Neighbour-Joining (N-J) tree computed on individual genetic distance showed that all Pentro young horses clustered together.

Keywords: pentro young horses, microsatellite, genetic distance

Introduction

The remains of an autochthonous horse population called "Cavallo Pentro" is bred in the wild in the mountainous area of the Molise region in Italy. The population is well adapted to the difficult environment of the "Pantano della Zittola", its breeding area. This is a wide plain located along the border of the Abruzzo National Park in the mountainous territory between the regions of Abruzzo and Molise. Living conditions in this area are very difficult because of the harsh climate; the winter is cold with floods and abudant snow while the summer is very dry. Moreover, the presence of predator, mainly wolves and bears from the nearby National Park, represent a constant danger for the livestock.

Historical informations about this population, together with morphological data and the genetic characterisation by microsatellite markers carried out on all the horses, adults and young horses were used, for the constitution of an "Anagraphic Register"of the "Pentro Horse" in the context of Italian equine autochthonous populations at extinction risk (Miraglia *et al.*, 2003). In this paper are reported data on genetic molecular analysis of the selected young horses according to the morphology.

Material and methods

Morphological and genealogical data were collected and blood samples were taken from a total of 23 Pentro young horses. In addition, six Italian horse breeds (Maremmano – 20 individuals, TPR – 20 individuals, Murgese – 20 individuals, Haflinger – 20 individuals, Trottatore – 20 individuals and Bardigiano – 20 individuals) were used as a comparison.

DNA samples were obtained from lymphocytes with the classical phenol-chloroform extraction protocol (Sambrook *et al.*, 1989).

Microsatellites genotypes were determined at each of twelve loci (HTG10, VHL20, HTG7, HTG4, AHT5, AHT4, HMS3, HMS6, HMS7, LEX003, HMS2, ASB2) for a total of 241 horses with a protocol of multiplex-PCR (Blasi *et al.*, 1999). For each locus the chromosomal location, the primer reference and size range in the studied populations are reported in Table1. Primer sequences and PCR amplification conditions are available from the authors. Genotypes were scored with an ABI PRISM 377 automatic sequencer and the GENESCAN and GENOTYPER computer packages.

Genetic distance by Nei (1987) was used for the breed comparison, while distances among individuals were calculated as the proportion of shared alleles, (Dps=1-Ps) according to Bowcock *et al.* (1994) using the MICROSAT program (Minch *et al.*, 1995). Neighbour-Joining diagram (Saitou *et al.*, 1987) were constructed on genetic distances using the PHYLIP package ver. 3.5c (Felsenstein, 1993). The program TreeView (Page, 1996) was used to visualize the diagram.

Table 1. References, chromosomal location and size range in base pair (bp) of the 12 microsatellite loci.

Locus	Reference	Chrom.	Size range (bp)
HTG10	Marklund *et al.*, 1994	21	88-116
VHL20	Van Hearingen *et al.*, 1992	30	87-107
HTG7	Marklund *et al.*, 1994	4	114-132
HTG4	Ellegren *et al.*, 1992	9	125-139
AHT5	Binns *et al.*, 1995	6	127-145
AHT4	Goddard *et al.*, 1998	24	146-164
HMS3	Guerin *et al.*, 1994	9	152-170
HMS6	Guerin *et al.*, 1994	4	157-171
HMS7	Guerin *et al.*, 1994	1	173-185
LEX03	Coogle *et al.*, 1996	X	195-217
HMS2	Guerin *et al.*, 1994	10	215-239
ASB2	Breen *et al.*, 1997	15	219-255

Results and discussion

In order to test the uniqueness of the selected offsprings, genetic distance among individuals were calculated as the proportion of shared alleles and used to build a N-J diagram. This method, proposed by Bowcock *et al.* (1994) for the study of human populations was recently used on horses as a statistical test for breed assignment (Bjornstad *et al.*, 2001). Bjornstad's study (2001) shows how 10 microsatellite markers are enough to give a result of a 75% in terms of correct assignment while raising the number of markers up to 20 increases the successful assignment to 95%.

The tree shows a high degree of structuring of the breeds. All the breeds display a good level of correct clustering (Figure 1). The Pentro horse group together in 100% of the cases. These results confirm the hypothesis of the Pentro horse being a genetic unit well differetiated from all the breeds analyzed in this work. This result is even more interesting if the introduction of genetic material from some of those breeds in the Pentro population is taken into account. The Pentro horse, despite all the foreign genetic material which has been introduced, has conserved its uniqueness. This introduction did not cause a total fading of the morphological characteristics of the original population.

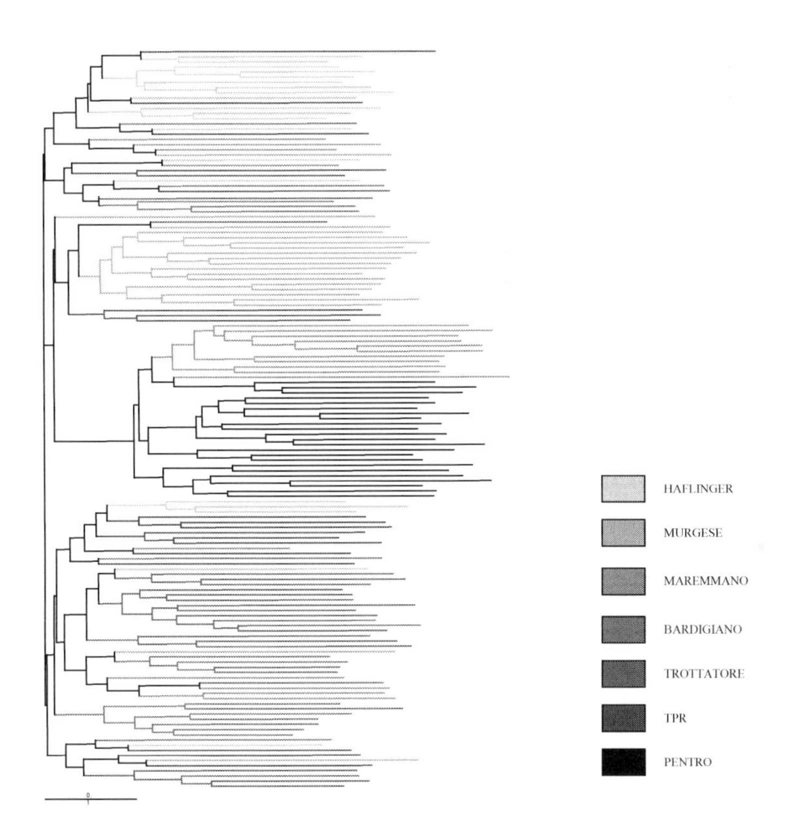

Figure 1. N-J diagram of distances among individuals constructed using the proportion of shared alleles.

Conclusions

Interbreeding is a common practice between the breeders and it is used to modify the characteristics of breeds according to the needs and also to expand the size of population when it is becoming too small. This practice is useful in a sense to preserve from excessive inbreeding, but it is also deleterious where small endagered populations are concerned. In this paper the case of the Pentro horse is presented, but other breeds seem to suffer from problems of this nature.

Molecular tool showed to be useful to assist the offsprings selection.

The uniqueness of the Pentro horse resides in its adaptive ability, which preserved it from complete "extinction" throught mixing with other breeds. The preservation of not only a natural, but also a social and cultural environment, is essential for the conservation of livestock genetic resources.

References

Bjornstad, G. and KH. Roed, 2001. Breed demarcation and potential for beed allocation of horses assessed by micrasatellite markers. Anim. Genet. 32: 59-65.

Blasi, M., A. Lanza, G. Perrotta and A. Rando, 1999. Evaluation of twelve microsatellites for parentage testing in trotter horses. in Proc. 13th Nat. Congr. ASPA, Piacenza, Italy, pp. 197-199.

Bowcock, AM., A. Ruiz-Linares, J. Tomfohrde, E. Minch, J.R. Kidd and LL. Cavalli-Sforza, 1994. High resolution of human evolutionary trees with polymorphic microsatellites. Nature. 368:455-457.

Breen, M., P. Downs, Z. Irvin and K. Bell, 1994. Intragenic amplification of horse microsatellite markers with emphasis on the Przewalski's horse (E. Przewalski), Anim. Genet. 25: 401-405.

Bruzzone, A., D. Iamartino, M. Blasi and F. Pilla, 2003. The Pentro horse: genetic characterisation by microsatellite markers. Ital. J. Anim. Sci. 2: 223-230.

Coogle, L., R. Reid and E. Baley, 1996. Equine dinucleotide repeat loci LEX015- LEX024. Anim. Genet. 27: 217-218.

Ellegren, H., M. Joansson, K. Sandberg and L. Andresson, 1992. Cloning of highly polymorphic microsatellites in the horse. Anim. Genet. 32: 133-142.

Felsenstein, J., 1993. PHYLIP (Phylogeny Inference Package). Version 3.5c distributed by the author. Departement of Genetics, University of Washington, Seattle, USA.

Godard, S., D. Vaiman, A. Oustry, M. Nocart, M. Bertaud, S. Guzylack, J.C. Meriaux, E.P. Cribiu and G. Guerin, 1997. Characterization genetic and physical mapping analysis of 36 horse plasmid and cosmid-derived microsatellites. Mamm. Gen. (8), 745-750.

Guerin, G., M. Bertaud and Y. Amigues, 1994. Characterisation of seven new horse microsatellites: HMS1, HMS2, HMS3, HMS4, HMS5, HMS6, HMS7 and HMS8. Anim. Genet. 25: 62.

Marklund, S., H. Ellegreen, S. Eriksson, K. Sandberg and L. Andersson, 1994. Parentage testing and linkage analysis in the horse using a set of highly polymorphic microsatellites. Anim. Genet. 25: 19-32.

Minch, E., A. Ruiz-Linares, D.B. Godstein, M.W. Feldman and L.L. Cavalli-Sforza, 1995. MICROSAT, A computer program for calculating various statistics on microsatellite alleli data (version 1.4d). Stanford University Medical Center.

Miraglia, N., F. Pilla, D. Gagliardi and M. De Renzis, 2003. Pentro horse: enrolment in the Anagraphic Register of the autochthonous equine populations. Proc. 5th *New findings in equine practice* Congr., Torino, Italy, pp 25-31.

Nei, M., 1987. Molecular evolutionary genetics. Columbia University Press, New York, USA.

Page, R.D.M., 1996. TreeView: an application to display phylogenetics trees on personal computer. CABIOS. 12: 357-358.

Sambrook, J., E.F. Fritsch and T. Maniatis, 1989. Molecular cloning: a laboratory manual. Cold Spring Harbor Laboratory Press, New York, USA.

Saitou, N. and M. Nei, 1987. The Neighbour-Joining method: a new method for reconstructing phylogenetics trees. Mol. Biol. Evol. 4: 406-425.

Van Haeringen, H., A.T. Bowling, M.L. Stott, J.A. Lenstra and K.A. Zwaagstra, 1994. A highly polymorphic horse microsatellite locus: VHL20. Anim. Genet. 25: 207.

The Retuertas horse: the "missing link" in the Iberoamerican horse breeds origin?

J.L. Vega-Pla[1]*, J. Calderón*[2]*, P.P. Rodríguez-Gallardo*[1]*, B. Alcaide*[1]*, F.T.P.S. Sereno*[3]*, M.R. Costa*[3]*, E. Pérez-Pineda*[4]*, A.M. Martínez*[5]*, J.V. Delgado*[5] *and C. Rico*[2]

[1]*Laboratorio de Genética Molecular, Servicio de Cría Caballar y Remonta, Aptdo. Oficial Sucursal 2, 14071-Córdoba, Spain*
[2]*Estación Biológica de Doñana, Pabellón del Perú, Sevilla, Spain*
[3]*Embrapa Amazonía Oriental, Belem-Pa, Brazil*
[4]*Universidad de Granma. Cuba*
[5]*Departamento de Genética, Universidad de Córdoba, Campus de Rabanales, Córdoba, Spain*

Introduction

The evolution of the horse can be traced through fossil remains to *Eohippus,* a small, leaf-browsing mammal of the Eocene. Several species and related genera appeared in North America and the Old World during the Eocene. For unknown reasons the Old World species went extinct, but the American species gave rise, in the Oligocene to the genus *Mesohippus.* During the Pleistocene the genus *Equus* apparently spread from North America to Asia and Europe via the Arctic-Asia land bridge. Then, suddenly, no one is absolutely certain why, between 10,000 and 8,000 years ago, *Equus* disappeared from North and South America. Various theories have been advanced to explain this extinction including destruction by drought, disease, or as a result of hunting by the recently arrived human populations. The fact is that the horse was gone from the western hemisphere by the time human civilizations were emerging in the eastern hemisphere. The submergence of the Bering land bridge prevented any migration from the Old World or Asia, and the horse was not seen again on its native continent until the Spanish explorers brought horses by ship in the sixteenth century.

The first arrival of modern horses to the American continent was in the first Columbus trip. Ten stallions and ten mares were included in this expedition. Columbus is know to have complained to King Ferdinand, he had paid for good horses, only to find that in his absence on the docks, peasant horses had been loaded on to his ships rather than the better stock for which he had paid. He wrote to the Catholic Monarch of Castilla: "*...you will tell their highnesses that as the keepers of horses came from Granada in the show made in Sevilla they rode good horses and after shipping I could not see them because I was a little ill and they gave us such animals that the best of them did not seem to cost more than 2000 Maravedies; they sold the goods and bought these...*" (Tudela, 1987). This may have been a lucky thing for the Spanish in some ways, for the indigenous Iberian horse stock probably had a higher survival rate during the voyages to the Americas than the larger and higher breed Andalusians.

On Spain's second voyage to the Americas in 1494 Columbus brought 24 stallions, 10 mares, 3 mules, 10 donkeys and an unspecified number of sheep and pigs to the island of Hispaniola. In 1511 a colony was established in Cuba, followed by Mexico, Puerto Rico, and Jamaica. Livestock was introduced in each of these American settlements. Spanish exports arrived directly from the ports of Spain to their final destination, with a stop on the Canary Islands or the Antilles.

The Colonial Spanish America was formed in three differentiated phases, playing the horses a different role in each of them. The first phase was the discovering where adventurers such as Columbus himself and his crew were responsible for the localization of new places and routes, the preparation of maps, and the location of new bases. In this phase the horses played a very marginal role, as they had no significant use in a phase based on navigation. The second phase was the conquest, in this case developed by soldiers who subjugated the native human populations and forced them to assimilate the rules, culture and religion of the Spaniards. In this phase the horse played a central role in the conquest of the entire continent as a war animal marking a huge difference between a western army with the native defences. Undoubtedly, the horses employed in the conquest sometime escaped during the battles or were robbed by native people promoting the formation of local horse populations, sometimes as domestics but also as feral animals. Up to this moment only pigs and chickens that were used as a food source accompanied the horses in the human activities (Delgado *et al.* 2004). The final phase was the colonization. This was developed by families that introduced to the American continent new animals (cattle, sheep and goats) but also more horses (for work), pigs and chickens. At the same time that the agriculture and other economic activities, performing the Creole society base of the present Latin American one (Rodero *et al.* 1992).

At the time of the American conquest, there were in Spain three main morphological equine types: the Celtic type of tarpanic origin in the north and west region of the peninsula; the Andalusian type (today known as Spanish Pure Breed), descendent from the African Barb horse and crossed with other European horses during XVI, XVII and XVIII centuries, in the south and east; and finally, in the central area, the hybrid between both of them. As Seville, Cadiz and other southern ports monopolized the navigation to America, it could be assumed that horses taken to America were mainly of the Spanish or Andalusian type (Rodero *et al.* 1992). But, which were the primitive Spanish horses introduced to Iberoamerica? Where do they came from and how do they look like? Usually, researchers have considered the old Andalusian horse as the primary source of horses introduced to America.

Among the likely source populations, we found a feral population of horses, which grazed in the Guadalquivir salt-marshes in what occupies today the Doñana National Park. These horses known as Retuertas horse (horse of the swamp) could represent the primitive animals shipped by Columbus, but probably also an ancestor of the present Spanish Pure Breed. Retuertas horse seems to be a candidate because morphological characters and genetic evidence (see below). It is believed that these horses survived in wild conditions because the swamps and bottomlands of the Guadlquivir and Guadiamar Rivers remained an inaccessible wilderness even when most of the country was already settled and cultivated, and therefore that is where the wild horses finally had to take refuge. To this day, the delta of the river Guadalquivir is home of a wilderness area and wildlife refuge. Other remains of indigenous Iberian wild horses of Spanish type are known in Portugal as Sorraia. However, it is also documented that other equine types were exported to America. For example, in 1508 the Spanish Crown authorized the transport of 40 horses from Castilla in the expedition organized by Alonso Ojeda and Diego de Nicuesa to Panama. The horses were of the Celtic type, small and resistant. It is also documented that many animals died during the 2-month trip, and other animals from the intermediate ports, Canary Islands or Antilles, could have replaced them.

According to historical records, Creole horses descend from Spanish horses introduced in 1493 to Santo Domingo and in 1583 to the Río de la Plata by Don Pedro de Mendoza (Dowdall, 1985). Many of these war horses escaped or were abandoned, and rapidly returned to a more primal state in inhabit harsh areas as the Pampa. For the next four centuries, the

Criollo breed adapted itself to the vast South American plains through the pitiless process of natural selection. This adaptation to the rude conditions of life was determined by selective factors acting on wild populations, which permitted them to develop qualities of physical hardiness and resistance to diseases. The indigenous people became riders upon contact with the Spanish military and colonialists, and began raising these horses in semi-liberty in the vast plains. They transformed the horse into their mode of transportation, their hunting or working companion and their partner in games.

Native North Americans quickly mastered these wild horses and developed great horsemanship skills, while in parts of the continent dominated by Spanish and Portuguese the horse remained mostly under the control of the conquerors and mestizos. It created a "way of life" that later on became known as cowboy, vaquero, charro, gaucho, etc. It shared a common culture and costumes along thousands of kilometres from Texas, New Mexico or California, to Patagonia. Spanish horses descendant's breeds are indeed a treasure of genetic wealth from a time long gone. Some of these Spanish descendant breeds are Argentinean Creole, Uruguayan Creole, Peruvian Paso, Paso Fino, Mangalarga, Marajoara, Mustang, Quarter Horse, Andinian horse, the Nordestino etc.

Although several studies have attempted to document more precisely the origin of the horses that were taken to America (Trommershausen-Bowling *et al.*, 1985; Kelly *et al.*, 2002; Mirol *et al.*, 2002), the fact is that several issues remain controversial. For example, studies based on blood groups, biochemical polymorphims and DNA markers showed a relationship among American horse breeds and Spanish Pure Breed (Rodríguez- Gallardo *et al.*, 1992). However strong genetic influence of Barb horse from the North of Africa has also been described. Is know that this breed never arrived directly to America, therefore it is necessary to find the remains of an Iberian horse that might be related to the Barb horse. Clearly, the only way to find out more about the origins of these horses beyond anecdotic theories is to compare their genetic structure at several neutral loci with other Iberian, European and North African breeds.

The advent of mitochondrial DNA analysis in population genetics during the 1980s produced a revolutionary change in historical, biogeographic and phylogenetic perspectives on intra- and interspecific genetic studies (Avise, 1994). Since then, it has been widely used to infer intra- and interspecific phylogenetic relationships. Mitochondrial DNA studies in horses have proved useful to characterize intrabreed variation (Kavar *et al.*, 1999; Kim *et al.*, 1999; Bowling *et al.*, 2000, Mirol *et al.*, 2002), although retention of high level of ancestral polymorphism due a complex multigeneration origin makes phylogenetic inference difficult (Vila *et al.*, 2001).

The availability of other genetic markers offers the opportunity to investigate of genetic relationships among breeds or populations, this information is useful for phylogenetic or biodiversity studies on populations. For this purpose, it is customary to use genetic markers such as protein and blood group polymorphisms or DNA markers. Generally, the approach for the genetic analysis of these data consists of calculating genetic distances and constructing trees. Over the last 10 years a wealth of diverse applications of these markers and particularly of microsatellite loci have been used to elucidate genetic relationships at all sorts of evolutionary levels (reviwed in D. B. Goldstein and C. Schlötterer, eds. Microsatellites: Evolution and Applications. Oxford University Press, Oxford).

In this chapter we present a summary of an ongoing research program developed by our team over the Retuertas horse, a feral horse population located in the protected area of Doñana in the South-Western Spain. We hypothesise that these horses might represent an ancestor of the Latin-American native breeds of Iberian origin.

This study begin with a morphological description of the Retuertas horse, showing the statistics on some morphological variables together with some pictures of these animal in their environment. Using the Iberoamerican Network on the Conservation of the Local Domestic Animal Biodiversity for the Sustainable Rural Development (CYTED Program) our team has begun an in depth study over the genetic characterisation and relationship among Latin American breeds and their possible ancestors in Spain and Portugal. Here we resenting a breed's dendrogram built from genetic distances of eighteen horse populations including four Latin American breeds of Iberian origin (Pantaneiro, Marajoara, Mangalarga, Criollo Cubano), and fourteen European, also a sample of donkey was included in the study to root the tree. It is important to point out that the data presented here are only preliminary as we are presently analysing samples of breeds from other countries of Latin America.

Morphological description of the Retuertas horse breed

These horses are slightly down of the mean size of the species, their body proportions are balanced and their front head profiles are slightly convex. The body of these animals is harmonic; it gives the population an elegant aspect with strong, rhythmic and elastic movements. Figure 1 shows in detail a representative animal of the population, all the characteristics mentioned here are illustrated in this picture.

The predominant coat colour of the population is bay but also grey is admitted; always the hair is fine and short.

In Table 1 we show a statistical description of this horse breed obtained from 25 horses randomly chosen of the whole population (16 Females and 9 males).

Table 1. Descriptive statistics by sex of the main zoometrical variables (in cm) in the Retuertas horse population.

Group of variables	Anatomic reference	Mean males (cm) and SD	Standard deviation males	Mean females (cm)	Standard deviation females
Heights	To the Neck	142.33	2.74	140.44	3.22
	To the middle of the back	135.25	3.58	134.25	4.45
	To the entry of the rump	139.25	4.65	139.75	4.27
	To the insertion of the tail	125.75	7.05	125.88	6.41
Lengths	Of the rump	48.63	2.33	48.50	2.00
	Of the head	49.44	2.07	48.80	1.32
Widths	Of the rump	45.63	3.34	49.25	1.77
	Of the head	24.56	1.31	20.80	1.01
Diameters	Longitudinal of the body	142.78	3.56	145.94	6.55
	Back-breast bone	65.44	2.30	66.94	2.29
	Transversal of the body	45.00	3.66	66.94	2.26
Perimeters	Rectum of the chest	171.75	7.11	174.81	5.17
	Cannon bone	18.22	0.95	17.55	0.91
	Hoof	34.23	1.32	32.64	1.02

The size of the head is balanced with the body, showing a mean length, its profile is slightly convex as we mentioned before. The ears are slightly short, mobile and well inserted. The front head is plane and not very wide. Eyes have an intense expression and the orbits are not prominent. The face is long with no prominent nostrils. Width and length of the neck is medium, well inserted and shows a slight arc in the top. The back is short to medium in length, strong and rounded. The shoulder is long and very well inclined with an open angel at the elbow giving the front limbs free and graceful movement. The chest and rib cage are wide, deep and well muscled. The bottom line of the barrel runs nearly horizontal. The loins are medium in length, broad and well muscled, and the croup is rounded and moderately sloped. He has a naturally low set tail. The long, muscular forearm is set forward to allow for a long, sloping shoulder. His knees are well defined and flat. The cannon bone is short with well-defined sinew. The hocks are distinct with prominent tendons, tight skin and with slightly more angle than other light saddle breeds. Again the cannon bone is short and all legs are refined and show adequate perimeter in relation to the size of the body. The hoofs are hard, rounded and of good size.

The behavioural characteristics of these animals are different when they are bred in feral to domestic conditions. In the past, it was quite, noble and rustic but in feral conditions it is very excitable at human presence and shows a difficult management (Figure 3). It shows harmonic and beautiful movements with intense elevation of the extremities, but also with moderated extensions what give long and rhythmic steps.

Interestingly, the appearance and morphology of these animals are very far from the current demands of Spanish horse breeders, for this reason the population is almost restricted to the preserved area of the Biological Reserve of Doñana, where it constitutes one more element in the ecosystem together with a wide natural fauna and other two domestic animals, the Marismeña Cattle and the Churro Lebrijano Sheep breed. Figure 2 shows a "troupe" of these horses in their environment.

At an expert's eyes, the morphological similarities between these animals with other Latin American breeds are quite evident. Among the breeds that clearly resemble these horses one can mention the North American Mustang, the Andinian horse, the Nordestino, Marajoara brasilian horses, and the Uruguayan and Argentinean Creole horses. All of them count with formal descriptions. However, a formal comparative analysis of zoometric characters awaits to be carried out. It is also worth mentioning that in the Iberian peninsula there is not any other similar population to the Retuertas horse, and perhaps only the Spanish pure breed shows some common characteristics such as the head profile.

Genetic characterisation of the Retuertas horse breed based on microsatellites

The Retuertas population has been forgotten by science and government institutions until recently, when a consortium formed by the Biological Reserve of Doñana, the University of Córdoba, and the Provincial Government of Córdoba begun an in depth study of this animal. Initially it was decided to perform a morphological description of the population, but the results promted us to formulate several new questions. Can this population be considered a zootechnical breed? Where do they come from? May have they participated in the origin of the Latin American Creole breeds? As mentioned above, only a genetic characterisation of these horses could potentially answer these and other questions. To this end, we carried out an extensive genetic study using protein and DNA polymorphism from 22 microsatellite loci. We choose microsatellites because they have proved to be the most informative genetic markers for elucidating population relationships in both, wild and domestic animals including horses (e.g. Moazami-Goudarzi *et al.*, 1997; McHugh *et al.*, 1998; Martínez *et al.*, 2000; Cañon *et al.*, 2000; Bjornstad *et al.*, 2002; Kelly *et al.*, 2002; Sereno, 2002).

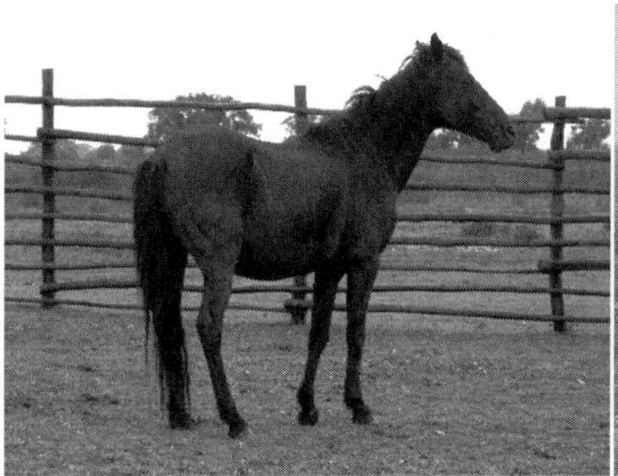

Figure 1. Representative animal of the Retuertas population kept in a fence for Taking the picture.

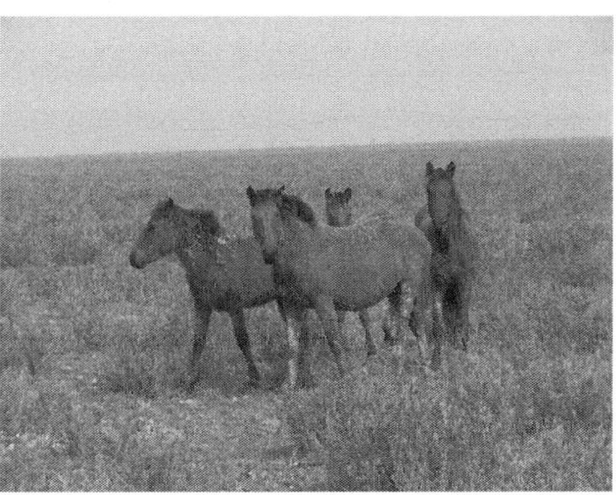

Figure 2. "Troupe" of animals in the Doñana Park Marshes. Observe the sand in the coat of the animals.

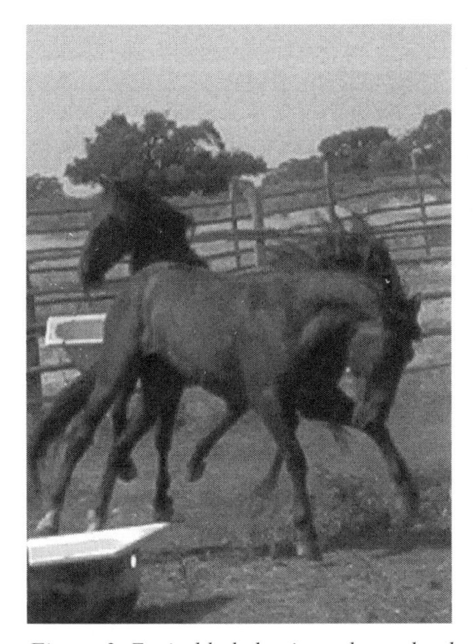

Figure 3. Excitable behaviour shown by these animals after housing.

In principle, it is easy to hypothesize that these horses should be closely related to other Iberian breeds of domestic animals or else to other European and/or North African breeds of Arabian-like horses that may have been introduced in large numbers during the middle-ages by the Moorish. Alternatively, an unlikely scenario would have been that these horses were descendants of a wild South Iberian population that have remained reproductively isolated due to limited individual dispersal and no selective breeding. This possibility was however, extremely remote, but there was nothing to loose in believing so.

In our study we have collected from the nucleus of this population breeding in the Doñana Biological Reserve 55 fresh blood samples of Retuertas horses (RET). Blood and hair samples from other 619 horses were randomly collected from thirteen breeds and distributed as follows (brackets show the breed's abbreviation and sample size): Spanish Pure Breed or Andalusian (60), Marismeño (26), Thoroughbred (46), Arabian (48); Celtic horses form the North of Spain as Losino (58), Asturcon (39) and Potok (27); Autochthonous horses from Balearic Islands: Mallorquin (30) and Menorquín (69); some Latin-American horse breeds as Cuban (24), Pantaneiro (45), Marajoara (60), Mangalarga (43), and Also donkey samples (*Equus asinus*) (44) were collected in order to use them as outgroup.

The DNA was extracted, PCR amplified for 22 microsatellite loci: AHT 4 and 5 (Binns *et al.*, 1995), ASB 2 and 17 (Breen *et al.*, 1997) ASB 23 (Lear *et al.*, 1999), HMS 3, 6 and 7 (Guerín *et al.*, 1994), HTG 4 (Ellegren *et al.*, 1992), HTG 10 (Marklund *et al.*, 1994), LEX 33 (Shiue *et al.*, 1999), TKY 279, 287, 294, 297, 301, 312, 321, 325, 333, 337 and 341 (Tozaky *et al.*, 2001). PCR products were separated by electrophoresis in an ABI 377 XL automatic sequencer (Applied Biosystems, Foster City, CA, USA). Bands were analysed using a Genescan v3.2.1 and Genotyper v2.5 software from the same manufacturer.

The results of this genotyping were subjected to a complete population genetic analysis and well as a phylogentic type analysis to elucidate the possible relationships with the other studied breeds.

In terms of genetic diversity we found a slight lower number of alleles in the Retuertas population with respect the other studied breeds. However this difference was negligible when the F statistics were calculated which was similar among the studied breeds. Furthermore, all comparisons between pairs of breeds gave fixation indices significantly different from zero. These figures indicate that all these breeds are well differentiated and there is little or no gene flow among them.

We have also determined that this breed is clearly differentiated of the other breeds in its context. The phenograms constructed with the Neighbour Joining algorithm using chord distance (D_{CE}) or Nei's distance (Da) or the maximum likelihood phenogram depicted four main clusters. The topology of these phenograms was identical and thus only the phenogram obtained with Da distance is presented. The unrooted neighbour-joining breed phenogram built from the obtained Da distances was rooted using donkey as outgroup (Figure 4). One cluster grouped Atlantic Celtic horses (Asturcon, Pottok and Losino), other cluster included Balearic Island breeds (Menorquin and Mallorquin). Brazilian breeds are clustered together and very well differentiated from Cuban horse. Finally, Arabian, Thoroughbred and Spanish Pure Breed are differentiated as expected Marismeño population is closely related with Spanish Pure Breed horse and as expected fall well in that fourth cluster. This is not surprising as the Marismeño population is often crossbred with Spanish Pure Breed stallions because the traditional breeding of this population. Interestingly the Retuertas population did not cluster with either of these four major clades and is located alone near of tree root. This result was the same independently of the method used to obtain the breed phenogram.

Although these results are only preliminary and cannot be taken as evidence for the relationship of the Retuertas horse as an ancestral population that was involved in the origin of the Spanish and Latin American horses they point out in this direction. The fact that the Retuertas population is recovered in the population dendrogram in a basal position suggests that it is ancestral to other European breeds. It is essential now to analyse several other Latin American and North African breeds to confirm of dismiss this hypothesis.

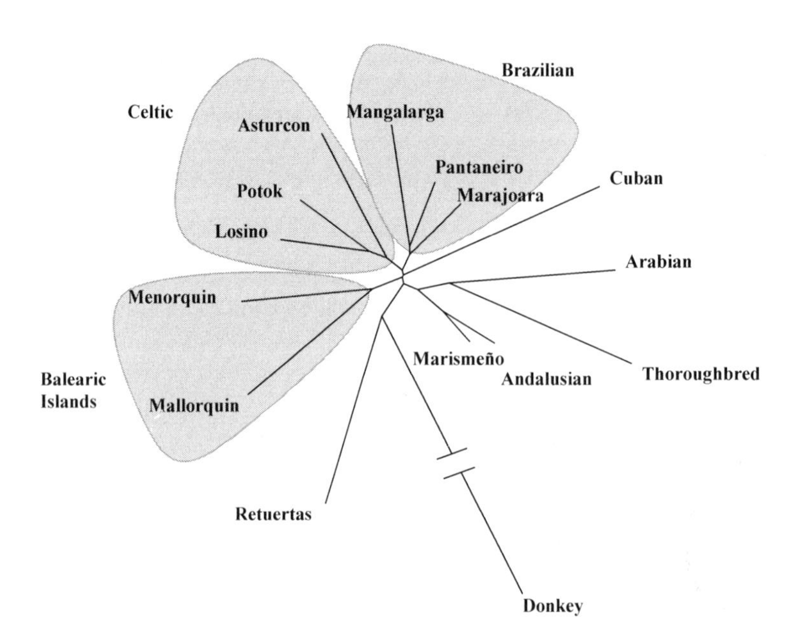

Figure 4. Neighbour-joining tree built from Da distances of eleven horse populations including a sample of donkey to root the tree.

A rare esterase allele as genetic marker of the Retuertas horse breed

The analysis of the biochemical polymorphism has been used in the past for studies of genetic characterization or genetic distancing among populations, but today this is almost completely replaced by molecular studies, specially the use of microsatellite typing. Even though, these methods conserve some relevance in the paternity verification procedures to compare genotypes with stallions and mares dead some years ago. In the Spanish official Studbook Laboratory typing serum allozyme biochemical polymorphis is still a routine task.

In this way, we have applied over 55 individuals of the Retuertas population an systematic analysis of A1B-Glycoprotein, Albumin, Carboxilesterase, Vitamin D-binding protein, Transferrin and Protein inhibitor variants using one-dimensional PolyAcrilamide Gel Electroforesis (PAGE) of plasma proteins according to Juneja and Gahne (1980).

Interestingly the Retuertas population showed an Esterase allele “L” that is very rare in Spanish Pure breed and practically do not appear in other breeds with exception of Barb horses (Ourag, 1994). It indicates a closed relationship between them.

Conclusions

1. The Retuertas horse population genetically different to the Spanish and other European horse breeds.
2. This population is a biological and zootechnical "jewel" that is needing a immediate intervention for its conservation because its small population size makes it particularly vulnerable. Its definitive administrative recognition as Spanish autochthonous breed is the first measure required.
3. The historical data, the geographical location and its basal position on a horse breed dendrograme suggest this population might well represent one of the ancestors of the present Latin American breeds. Although, this relation has to be demonstrated the evidence so far suggest that it is the missing link between Barb, Spanish Pure Breed and American Horses.

References

Binns, M, J.E. Swinburne and M. Breen, 2000. Molecular genetics of the horse. In: A.T. Bowling and A. Ruvinsky, The genetics of the horse. New York: CABI Publishing, p.109-121.

Bjornstad, G. and K.H. Roed, 2002. Evaluation of factors affecting individual assignment precision using microsatellite data from horse breeds and simulated breed crosses. Animal Genetics, v.33, 264-270, 2002.

Bowling, A.T., M.L. Eggleston-Stott, G. Byrns, R.S. Clark, S. Dileanis and E. Wictum, 1997. Validation of microsatellite markers for routine horse parentage testing. Animal Genetics, v.28, p.247-252.

Breen, M., G. Lindgren, M.M. Binns, J. Norma, Z. Irvin, K. Bell, K. Sandberg and H. Ellegren, 1997. Genetical and physical assignments of equine microsatellites - First integration of anchored markers in horse genome mapping. Mammalian Genome, v.8, p.267-273.

Cañon, J., M.L. Checa, C. Carleos, J.L. Vega-Pla, M. Vallejo and S. Dunner, 2000. The genetic structure of Spanish Celtic horse breeds inferred from microsatellite data. Animal Genetics, v.31, p.39-48.

Delgado, J.V., M.E. Camacho, J.M. León, M.R. de la Haba, A. Vallecillo, C. Barba and A. Cabello, 2004. Poblaciones Porcinas en Iberoamérica. In: Biodiversidad Porcina Iberoamericana: Caracterización y usos sustentables (Ed J.V. Delgado) p.21-31. Ed. Universidad de Córdoba, Spain.

Ellegren, H., M. Johansson, K. Sandberg and L. Andersson, 1992. Cloning of highly polymorphic microsatellites in horse. Animal Genetics, v.23, p.133-142.

Guérin, G., M. Bertand and Y. Amigues, 1994. Characterisation of seven new horse microsatellites: HMS1, HMS2, HMS3, HMS5, HMS6, HMS7, HMS8. Animal Genetics, v.25, p.62.

Kelly L., A. Postiglioni, D.F. De Andres, J.L. Vega-Pla, R. Gagliardi, R. Biagetti and J. Franco, 2001. Genetic Characterisation of the Uruguayan Creole Horse and analysis of relationships among horse breeds. Research in Veterinary Science, v.72, p.69-73.

Lear, T.L., R. Brandon and K. Bell, 1999. Physical mapping of ten equine dinucleotide repeat microsatellites. Animal Genetics, v.30, p.235.

Luís, C., C. Bastos-Silveira, E.G. Cothran, M.M. Oom,. Iberian and new world horse breeds: do they show phylogenetic relationship? Abstracts of IV Congreso Ibérico de la Sociedad de Recursos Genéticos Animales. p.364

Marklund, S., H. Ellegren, S. Eriksson, K. Sandberg and L. Andersson, 1994. Parentage testing and linkage analysis in the horse using a set of highly polymorphic microsatellites. Animal Genetics, v.25, p.19-23.

Martínez, A.M., J.V. Delgado, A. Rodero and J.L. Vegla-Pla, 2000. Genetic structure of the Iberian pig breed using microsatellites. Animal Genetics, v.30, p.177-182.

McHugh, D.E., R.T. Loftus, P. Cunningham and D.G. Bradley, 1998. Genetic structure of seven European cattle breeds assessed using 20 microsatellite markers. Animal Genetics, v.29, p.333-340.

Mirol, P.M., P. Peral García, J.L. Vega-Pla, F.N. Dulot, 2002. Phylogenetic relationships of Argentinean Creole horses and other South American and Spanish breeds inferred from mitochondrial DNA sequences. Animal Genetics v.33, p.356-363.

Moazami-Goudarzi, K., D. Laloë and J.P. Furet, 1997. Grosclaude, F. Analysis of genetic relationships between 10 cattle breeds with 17 microsatellites. Animal Genetics, v.28, p.338-345.

Nei, M., 1983. Genetic polymorphism and the role of mutation in evolution. In: M. Nei and. R. Khoen (Ed.) Evolution of genes and proteins, 165-190, Sunderland.

Ouragh, L., J.C. Mériaux and J.P. Braun, 1994. Genetic Blood markers in Arabian, Barb and Arab-Barb horses in Morocco. Animal Genetics v.25, p.45-47.

Rodero, A., J.V. Delgado and E. Rodero, 1992. Primitive Andalusian livestock and their implication in the discovery of America. Archivos de Zootecnia, v.41, p.383-400.
Rodriguez-Gallardo, P.P., P. Aguilar, J.L. Vega-Pla and D.F. De Andres, 1992. Blood group and polymorphism gene frequencies for the Andalusian Horse breed. A comparison with four American Horse breeds. Archivos de Zootecnia, v.41, p.433-442.
Saitou, N. and M. Nei, 1987. The neighbour-joining method: a new method for reconstructing phylogenetic trees. Molecular Biology and Ecology. v.4, p.406-25.
Sereno, F.T.P.S., 2002. Caracterización genética del caballo Pantaneiro. Thesis doctoral. Cordoba University. Spain.
Shiue, Y.-L., L.A. Bickel, A.R. Caetano, L.V. Millon, R.S. Clark, M.L. Eggleston, R. Michelmore, E. Bailey, G. Guérin, S. Godard, J.R. Mickelson, S.J. Valberg, J.D. Murray and A.T. Bowling, 1999. A synteny map of the horse genome comprised of 240 microsatellite and RAPD markers. Animal Genetics, v.30, p.1-9.
Tackezaki, N. and M. Nei, 1996. Genetic distances and reconstruction of phylogenetic trees from microsatellite DNA. Genetics, v.144, p.389-399.
Tozaki, T., H. Kakoi, S. Mashima, K. Hirota, T. Hasegawa, N. Ishida, N. Miura, N.H. Choi-Miura and M. Tomita, 2001. Population study and validation of paternity testing for Thoroughbred horses by 15 microsatellite loci. Journal Veterinary Medicine Science, v.63, p.1191-1197.
Trommershausen-Bowling, A. and R.S. Clark, 1985. Blood group and protein polymorphism gen frequencies for seven breeds of horses in the United States. Anima blood Groups and Biochemical Genetics v.16, p.93-104.
Tudela, 1987. El legado de España a América. Vol II. Ed. Pegaso. Madrid.

Genetic diversity of the Zemaitukai Horse

R. Juras[1,2] *and E.G. Cothran*[2]

[1]*Siauliai University, Visinskio 25, LT-5400 Siauliai, Lithuania*
[2]*University of Kentucky,Department of Veterinary Science, Lexington, 40546-0099, KY, USA*

Abstract

A program for the preservation of the genetic resources of different farm animals was developed in Lithuania and includes the Zemaitukai horse, which is one of the native Lithuanian horses. In this study a wide range of genetic markers (12 microsatellites, 7 blood group loci, 10 biochemical loci) and mitochondrial DNA (mtDNA) sequencing were used to access genetic diversity in Zemaitukai horses. High levels of genetic variation for both genomic and mitochondrial DNA within the Zemaitukai horse breed was observed. Based on genetic distance values, Zemaitukai do not show close relationship to any breed that we have tested, except for those of other Lithuanian horse breeds.

Keywords: conservation, diversity, genetic distance, genetic variation, horse

Introduction

Domesticated animals in the last hundred years have been subjected to great pressure to evolve to meet the changing needs of a commercialized, mechanized and globalized world. Today a large number of the world's breeds are in danger of extinction. As happened with breeds of other domestic species, some horse breeds are threatened by extinction because they do not appear to meet the current needs of humans. The Zemaitukai is an ancient indigenous Lithuanian horse breed. Throughout history, the role of Zemaitukai horse has changed from that of an excellent military horse during the Lithuanian-Crusader Battles to an all-purpose utility horse. As a consequence of unfavorable historical and economical circumstances as well as disorganized breeding work the number of Zemaitukai seriously declined, reduced to the lowest numbers in the breed history with 30 individuals left in 1994. The critical status was recognized and efforts for breed conservation from complete extinction were undertaken. The development of the conservation program plan, breed monitoring, formation of the breeding herds and studies of the biological and farming qualities of the horses were begun in 1994 (Garbacauskaite, 1998). In order to minimize the effect of inbreeding crossbreeding was used. Estonian native and Polish primitive (Konik) horses were used. Only crossbreeding with Estonian native horses was successful. According to pedigree data, the Zemaitukai horse population consists of two stallion (male) and five mare (female) family lines (Macijauskiene, 2002). In the beginning of 2004 the Zemaitukai horse population consisted of 22 stallions, 67 mares and 57 breeding progeny (Macijauskiene, 2004).

Biological reasons for conservation, such as genetic insurance or scientific value, are important as well as historical and cultural reasons for conserving genetic resources. A correct pedigree is important for any domestic horse breed whether rare or not. For breeds that are common, an incorrect pedigree can frustrate breeding plans for selective improvement of the breed. For rare breeds, correct pedigrees are important for developing breeding strategies that minimize inbreeding. Genetic marker analysis is useful for determining the current genetic status of the population and also can be used as a management tool for maintenance of small populations (maintaining genetic variability). Genetic markers could be used to determine relationship with other populations and comparative genetic analysis could provide input into a rare breed conservation management plan. Genetic variation within a breed can be divided into two components: a) populational genetic diversity and b) individual genetic variance. Reduction of the populational genetic diversity can result in the loss of long-term adaptability and survival probability of the breed. Loss of individual variation, mainly due to inbreeding, can cause a reduction in individual fertility and viability. It is important to evaluate the amount of genetic variability still present in horse populations in order to develop better conservation programmes. Genetic markers designed for parentage verification (blood groups, microsatellites) have been extensively used to assess levels of genetic variation of different horse populations, to compare populations and, to determine relationships with other populations (e.g. Cothran *et al.*, 1998, Cannon *et al.*, 2000; Juras *et al.*, 2003 Tozaki *et al.*, 2003). Like the genomic DNA, mitochondrial DNA is useful for studying the evolution of closely related species. Mitochondrial DNA sequence polymorphism has been used to examine genetic relationship within breeds (Hill *et al.*, 2002; Luis *et al.*, 2002), among breeds (Kim *et al.*, 1999; Mirol *et al.*, 2002), between domestic and wild horse populations (Oakenfull & Ryder, 1998) and also to address questions of horse domestication (Lister *et al.*, 1998; Vila *et al.*, 2001).

Material and methods

Blood samples (n = 30) of Zemaitukai horses were collected by jugular venipuncture in acid-citrat-dextrose (ACD). The samples were separated into red blood cells (rbc), rbc lysate, and serum. DNA was extracted from whole blood with the Puregene DNA Extraction Kit (Gentra Systems, USA) following the manufacturer instructions. Standard immunological procedures involving hemaaglutination and complement mediated hemolysis (Stormont & Suzuki 1964; Stormont *et al.*, 1964) were used to detect variation of red cell alloantigens at seven blood group loci. Starch and polyacrylamide gel electrophoresis and isoelectric focusing were used to detect variation at 10 serum and rbc lysate protein loci (Braend, 1973; Sandberg, 1974; Junea, 1978; Braend & Johansen, 1983). The horse blood group loci analyzed were EAA, EAC, EAD, EAK, EAP, EAQ and EAU, and the biochemical protein loci were alpha-1-beta glycoprotein (A1β), albumin (ALB), serum esterase (ES), vitamin D binding protein (GC), glucosephosphate isomerase (GPI), alpha-heamoglobin (HBA), 6-phosphogluconate dehydrogenase (6-PGD), phosphoglucomutase (PGM), protease inhibitor (PI) and transferin (TF). Nomenclature for variants at all 17 loci was in accordance with internationally standardized usage for horses (Bowling & Clark, 1985; Bowling & Ryder, 1987) except for variants at some loci, which have not yet received international recognition.

The DNA typing panel consisted of 12 microsatellites: AHT4 and AHT5 (Binns *et al.*, 1995), ASB2 (Breen *et al.*, 1996), HMS2, HMS3, HMS6 and HMS7 (Guérin *et al.*, 1994), HTG4 and HTG6 (Ellegren *et al.*, 1992), HTG7 and HTG10 (Marklund *et al.*, 1994) and VHL20 (Van Haeringen *et al.*, 1994). Amplification of microsatellites in multiple PCR reactions was performed in 25μl total volume reactions containing 50 ng of genomic DNA, 0.07 to 0.8 pmol of primers, 1xPCR buffer (Perkin Elmer), 2.5mM $MgCl_2$, 0.2 mM dNTPs and lU AmpliTaq. For microsatellite amplification, a hot start procedure was used in which DNA template and primers were combined and heated at 95 °C for 10 min. The temperature was then lowered and held at 85 °C for 10 minutes for addition of the remaining reagents. 32 cycles of 1 minute at 95 °C, annealing 58 °C for 30 seconds and 72 °C for 45 seconds, then cycling was completed with a final extension at 72 °C for 30 min. Reaction products were analyzed using ABI 377 DNA sequencer (Applied Biosystems, Foster City, CA, USA). Fragment sizes were determinated using the computer software STRand (Hughes, 2000).

For mtDNA sequencing, primers from published horse mtDNA sequence (Xu and Arnason, 1994) were designed: Forward 5'-CGCACATTACCCTGGTCTTG-3', Reverse 5'-GAACCAGATGCCAGGTATAG-3'. Polymerase chain reaction (PCR) was carried out in 25 μl total reaction volumes, each containing 0.2 mM dNTP's, 0.5 μM of each primer, 2.5 mM $MgCl_2$, 1xPCR buffer, 1 U of Taq polymerase (PE Applied Biosystems, MA), 1U of AmpliTaq Gold (PE Applied Biosystems, MA) and 50 ng of template DNA. The reaction mixture was heated to 95 °C for 5 minutes, followed by 30 cycles each consisting of 40 seconds denaturation at 94 °C, 45 seconds annealing at 55 °C, 45 seconds of extension at 72 °C and then a final 10 minutes extension at 72 °C. Sequencing was carried out using BigDye™ Terminator Cycle Sequencing Kit (PE Applied Biosystems, MA). Sequences were determined using the ABI Prism 377 DNA Sequencer. All sequences were confirmed by re-sequencing the same sample using a second independent PCR reaction.

Gene frequencies for biochemical loci were calculated by direct count. Frequencies of alleles at blood group loci were calculated by the allocation method of Andersson (1985). Genetic variation was measured by the observed heterozygosity (Ho), Hardy-Weinberg expected heterozygosity (He), unbiased expected heterozygosity (Hu) Nei (1978), effective number of alleles (Ae), and the total number of variants found in each population (Na). In addition, population inbreeding level was estimated by Wright's Fis = 1 – (Ho/He). Values of genetic variation at blood group and biochemical loci of Zemaitukai horses were compared to those of 122 domestic horse populations that have been tested at the University of Kentucky and to 52 breeds at microsatellite loci (Cothran, E.G. unpublished results). A dendogram of genetic relationship was constructed using neighbour joining method (Takezaki and Nei, 1996).

Results and discussion

Measures of genetic variability at blood group and biochemical loci for the Zemaitukai horse population are given in Table 1. Variability values for other domestic horse breeds and the means of these measures based on data from 122 domestic horse breeds examinated at the University of Kentucky also are shown in Table 1. The breeds were selected to demonstrate the range of variability in the domestic breeds. There were no statistically significant deviations from expected levels of heterozygosity (based upon Hardy-Weinberg equilibrium theory) for any of the biochemical loci were Ho could be calculated. Individual genetic variation within the Zemaitukai was higher than the mean Ho for 122 domestic horse populations (Table 1). Of the 122 populations of domestic breeds that have been examined, only 12 have higher values of Ho than Zemaitukai. Thus, from a genetic conservation standpoint there is no immediate concern about reduced genetic variation within the Lithuanian horse breed. For populational variation measures the Zemaitukai had higher He and lower Ae and Na compared to the domestic horse mean (Table 1).

Table 1. Estimates of genetic variability for Zemaitukai and other selected domestic horse breeds at biochemical loci. The means of the genetic variation measures were based on data from 122 domestic horse populations. See text for variable definitions.

Breed	N	Ho	He	Hu	Fis	Na	Ae
Zemaitukai	30	0.430	0.377	0.384	-0.155	54	2.159
Thoroughbred	265	0.294	0.288	0.289	-0.019	64	2.009
Arabian	117	0.307	0.327	0.328	0.061	67	2.132
Exmoor pony	101	0.451	0.467	0.469	0.033	65	2.523
Skyros pony	79	0.434	0.418	0.420	-0.046	68	2.435
Konik	207	0.413	0.405	0.406	-0.021	68	2.544
Lipizzaner	98	0.355	0.324	0.325	-0.034	69	2.396
Haflinger	161	0.405	0.412	0.413	0.016	69	2.704
Quarter horse	168	0.396	0.393	0.394	-0.007	87	2.653
Suffolk punch	122	0.438	0.432	0.434	-0.013	65	2.459
Domestic horse mean	122	0.371	0.365	0.371	-0.015	65.11	2.390
Standard deviation		0.048	0.043	0.043	0.065	11.04	0.250

Lower values for the total number of alleles and effective number of alleles may be partly due to a small sample size. For this indigenous breed Ho exceeded He, resulting in negative Fis values. Considerably less variation in allele numbers and heterozygosity levels was detected in biochemical systems than microsatellites. This observation is in accordance with previous studies (e.g. Bjornstad *et al.*, 2000). At twelve microsatellite loci observed heterozygosity for Zemaitukai was slightly above the mean for domestic horse breeds (0.682 compare to 0.699). The values for expected heterozygosity and effective number of alleles were lower than those of the domestic horse mean (Table 2). The analysis of variation at the combined biochemical and microsatellite data sets was consistent with a bottleneck which fits the breed history of 1994. High levels of genetic variability found in Lithuanian horse breeds is similar to those of other studies carried out on rare breeds. High levels of variability have been found in rare breeds like the Posavina heavy horse breed from Croatia, Pantaneiro horse of Brazil, Chilote horse from Chile and others (Cothran *et al.*, 1993, Cotran & Kovac, 1997, Cothran *et al.*, 1998). The reasons why these rare breeds did not show reduced variation were not clear. Possibly, the reductions in population size were too recent to have resulted in reduced variation.

The analysis of mitochondrial DNA of Zemaitukai horses adds useful information for the effective management and conservation of this rare breed. Five different haplotypes were found for the five maternal lines of the Zemaitukai, confirming the pedigree information. The mtDNA results confirm the maternal lineages, from the pedigrees. This information is useful for development of breeding strategies aimed at evening the genetic contribution of different maternal founding lineages. The mtDNA data also provides additional insights into the genetic diversity of the breed, which, in combination with data from nuclear genes, can be used to maximize the maintenance of genetic diversity within the rare horse breeds.

Genetic relationship among horse breeds using restricted maximum likelihood analysis of the gene frequency data (blood group and biochemical loci) paired Zemaitukai and heavy type Zemaitukai (another Lithuanian breed) together, along with the Skyros pony from Greece, between clusters of Arabian type horses and Iberian type horse breeds (data not shown). Close relationship of Lithuanian horses to this indigenous Greek horse breed is very unlikely, it also is unlikely that Lithuanian horses actually share close ancestors with Arabian and Iberian type horse breed. Several other horse breeds from the same geographical region like Polish primitive horse (Konik), Hucul, Wielkopolski, and Finn horse failed to show close relationship to Lithuanian horse breeds. In a phylogenetic tree built with the neighbour joining method from microsatellite data, three Lithuanian horse breeds (the third is the Lithuanian Heavy Draught horse) were paired together with a closer relationship of Zemaitukai and heavy type Zemaitukai horses, which is the expected result (Figure 1).

Table 2. Estimates of genetic variability at microsattelite loci for Zemaitukai and other selected horse breeds. The means of the genetic variation measures were based on data from 51 domestic horse populations See text for variable definitions.

Breed	N	Ho	He	Hu	Fis	Na	Ae
Zemaitukai	30	0.682	0.641	0.651	-0.048	60	3.042
Thoroughbred	175	0.674	0.693	0.695	0.027	75	3.622
Arabian	93	0.625	0.681	0.687	0.072	78	3.657
Exmoor pony	98	0.601	0.606	0.609	0.014	63	2.733
Skyros pony	47	0.644	0.640	0.647	-0.010	62	3.153
Konik	150	0.674	0.668	0.673	0.005	74	3.597
Lipizzaner	77	0.687	0.717	0.723	0.068	81	3.610
Haflinger	341	0.630	0.639	0.641	0.017	75	3.264
Quarter horse	47	0.645	0.640	0.647	0.057	69	3.153
Suffolk punch	122	0.684	0.713	0.717	0.043	79	3.795
Domestic horse mean	51	0.699	0.698	0.711	0.015	75.39	3.767

The phylogenetic tree obtained from microsatellite data formed clusters according to breed type or relationship with only few exceptions. Further investigations of breeds from the same geographical area would contribute for better understanding of Lithuanian native horse breed origin and genetic relationship with other domestic horse breeds.

Due to historical circumstances, major population reductions, disorganized breeding work and economical circumstances led Zematukai horses to be at risk of disappearing. The conservation program was introduced in 1994 and the population was rebuilt after this critical period starting with 30 adults and 12 progeny horses. In order to avoid inbreeding and extend stallion lines crossbreeding was used in this breed, which probably contributed to high levels of genetic variation observed in this rare breed. Total size of the Zemaitukai horse population now is 149 individuals with the effective population number (Ne) of 66.9 based upon sex ratio (Macijauskiene, 2004); those figures, from the theoretical standpoint, are adequate for short-term maintenance only. However, based upon the known number of founders (as confirmed by mtDNA) Ne could be as low as 9. Although levels of variation are high, the small population size and limited founder numbers mean that diversity could decline rapidly. In order to maintain levels of genetic variation in the Zemaitukai horse a population monitoring program should be implemented. All animals before being accepted into stud books should be blood typed or DNA typed to check if the pedigree is correct, that will also allow to monitor levels of genetic variation in the population. The stud book should be closed in order to maintain uniqueness of the breed.

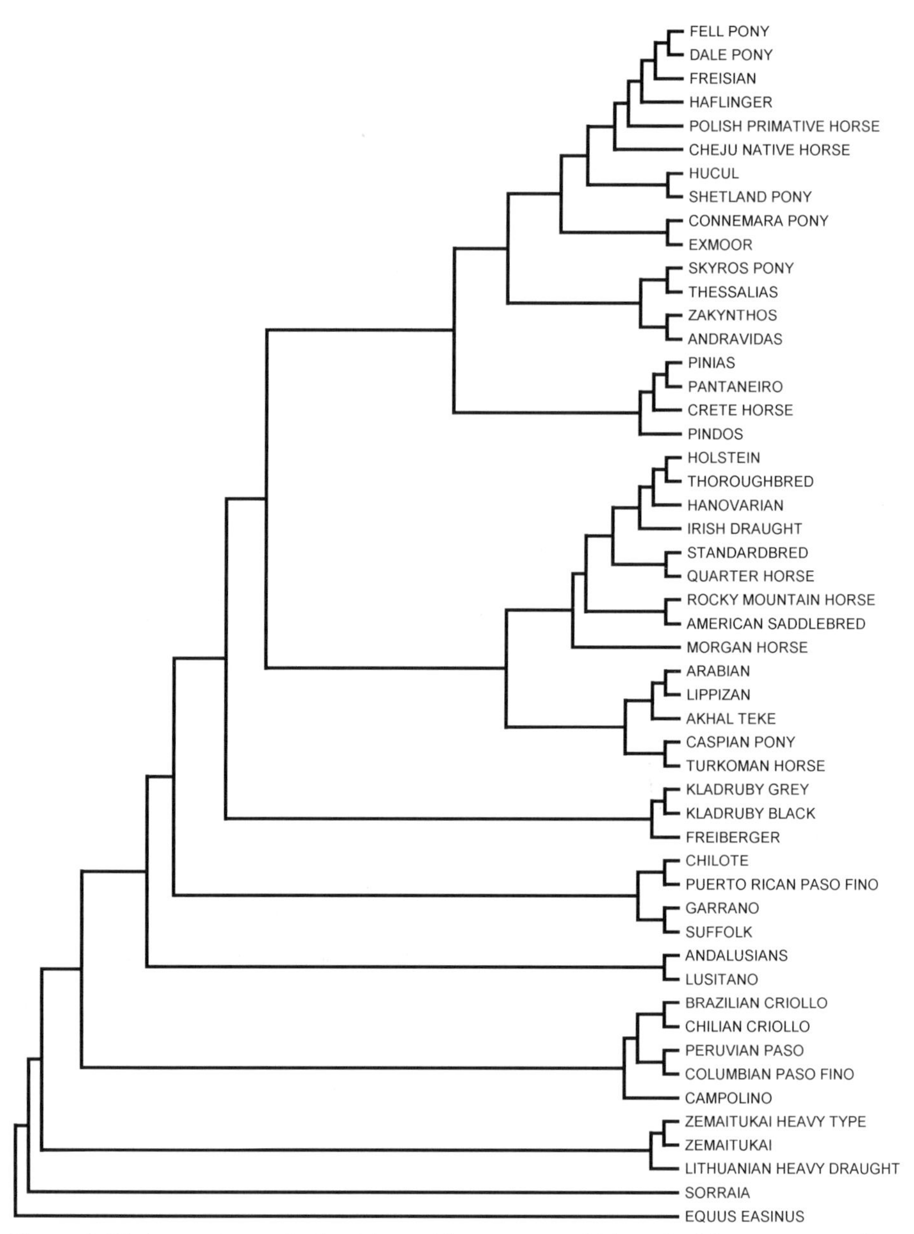

Figure 1. Phylogenetic tree built with neighbour joining (NJ) method from microsatellite data using donkey (Equus easinus) as outgroup.

References

Andersson, L., 1985. The estimation of blood group gene frequencies: a note on the allocation method. Anim. Blood Groups Biochem. Genet. 16, 1-7.
Binns, M.M., N.G. Holmes, A. Holliman and A.M. Scott, 1995. The identification of polymorphic microsatellite loci in the horse and their use in thoroughbred parentage testing. British Vet. J. 151, 9-15.
Bjornstad, G., E. Gunby and K.H. Roed, 2000. Genetic structure of Norwegian horse breeds. J.of Anim. Breeding and Gen. 117, 307-317.
Bowling, A.T. and O.A. Ryder, 1987. Genetic studies of blood markers in Przewalski's horse. Heredity 78, 75-80.
Bowling, A.T. and R.S. Clark, 1985. Blood group and protein polymorphism frequencies for seven breeds of horses in the United States. Anim. Blood Groups Biochem. Genet. 16, 93-108.
Braend, M. and K.E. Johansen, 1983. Haemoglobin types in Norwegian horses. Anim. Blood Groups Biochem. Genet. 14, 305-307.
Braend, M., 1973. Genetic variation in equine blood proteins. Karger, Basel, 394-406.
Breen, M., G. Lindgren, M.M. Binns, J. Norman, Z. Irvin, K. Bell, K. Sandberg and H. Ellegren, 1997. Genetical and physical assignments of equine microsatellites-first integration of anchored markers in horse genome mapping. Mammalian Genome 8, 267-273.
Canon, J., M.I. Checa, C. Carlos, J.L. Vega-Pla and S. Dunner, 2000. The genetic structure of Spanish horse breeds inferred from microsatellite data. Anim. Genet. 31, 39-48.
Cothran, E.G. and E. Van Dyk, 1998. Genetic analysis of three South African horse breeds. J. of South African Vet. Assoc. 69, 120-125
Cothran, E.G. and M. Kovac, 1997. Genetic analysis of the Croatian Trakehner and Posavina horse breeds. Zivocysna Vyroba. 5, 207-212.
Cothran, E.G., R. Mancilla, J. Oltra and M.V. Ortiz, 1993. Analysis genetico del caballo Chilote de la Isla de Chiloe-Chile. Archivos de Med.Vet. 2, 137-146.
Cothran, G.E., S.A. Santos, M.C.M. Mazza, T.L. Lear and J.R.B. Sereno, 1998. Genetics of the Pantaneiro horse of the Pantanal region of Brazil. Genet Mol. Biol.Vol. 21, 343-349.
Ellegren, H., M. Johansson, K. Sandberg and L. Andersson, 1992. Cloning of highly polymorphic microsatellites in the horse. Anim. Genet. 23, 133-42.
Garbacauskaite, V. 1998. The Zemaitukai horse breed and conservation of it's genopool. Lithuanian Institute of Animal Science. Doctoral dissertation. Baisogala. P. 23-32. (in Lithuanian).
Guerin, G., M. Bertaud and Y. Amiques, 1994. Characterization of seven new horse microsatellites: HMS1, HMS2, HMS3, HMS5, HMS6, HMS7 and HMS8. Anim. Genet. 25, 62.
Hill, E.W., D.G. Bradley, M. Al-Barody, O. Ertugul, R.L. Splan, I. Zakharov and E.P. Cunningam, 2002. History and integrity of thoroughbred dam lines revealed in the equine mtDNA variation. Anim. Genet. 33, 287-294.
Hughes S.S. 1.2.90. "Strand Nucleic Acid Analysis Software". Available: http://www.vgl.ucdaviess.edu/STRand. Univ. of Calif., Davies, CA. 2000.
Junea, R.K., B. Gahna and K. Sandberg, 1978. Genetic polymorphism of the Vitamin D binding protein and other post-albumin protein in horse serum. Anim. Blood Grps. Biochem. Genet. 25, 29-36.
Juras, R., E.G. Cothran and R. Klimas, 2003. Genetic analysis of three Lithuanian native horse breeds. Acta Agric. Scand., Sec. A., Animal Sci. 53, 180-185.
Kim, K.I., Y.H. Yang, S.S. Lee, C. Park, R. Ma, J.L. Bouzat and H.A. Lewin, 1999. Phylogenetics relationship of Cheju horses to other horse breeds as determined by mtDNA D-loop sequence polymorphism. Anim. Genet. 30, 102-108.
Lister, A.M., M. Kadwell, L.M. Kaagan, W.C. Jordan, M.B. Richards and H.F. Stanley, 1998. Ancient and modern DNA in study of horse domestication. Ancient Biomol. 2, 267-280.
Luís, C., C. Bastos-Silveira, E.G. Cothran and M.M. Oom, 2002. Mitochondrial control region sequence variation between the two maternal lines of the Sorraia horse breed. Genet. Mol. Biol. 25, 131-134.
Macijauskiene, V., 2002. Monitoring of the Zemaitukai horse breed. Anim. Husb. 40, 3-12.
Macijauskiene, V., 2004. Changes in size, value and structure of Zemaitukai horse population under conservation programme. X BABC, 183-187.
Marklund, S., H. Ellegren, S. Eriksson, K. Sandberg and L. Andersson, 1994. Parentage testing and linkage analysis in the horse using a set of highly polymorphic microsatellites. Anim. Genet. 25, 19-23.
Mirol, P.M., P. Peral Garcia, J.L. Vega-Pla and F.N. Dulout, 2002. Phylogenetic relationship of Argentinean Creole horses and other South American and Spanish breeds inferred from mitochondrial DNA sequences. Anim. Genet. 33, 356-363.
Nei, M., 1978. Estimation of average heterozigosity and genetic distance from a small number of individuals. Genetics 89, 583-590.
Oakenfull, E.A. and O.A. Ryder, 1998. Mitochondrial control region and 12S rRNR variation in Przewalski horse (*Equus przewalski*). Anim. Genet. 29, 456-459.

Rodgers, J.S., 1972. Measures of genetic similarity and genetic distance. Stud. Gene. VII Univ. Texas Publ. 7213, 145-153.
Sandberg, K., 1974. Blood typing of the horse: Current status and application to the identification problems. In: Proceedings of the 1st World Congress of Genetics Applied to Livestock Production. Madrid. 253-265.
Stormont, C. and Y. Suzuki, 1964. Genetic polymorphism of blood groups in horses. Genetics 50, 915-929.
Stormont, C., Y. Suzuki and E.A. Rhode, 1964. Serology of horse blood groups. Cornell Vet. 54, 439-452.
Takezaki, N. and M. Nei, 1996. Genetic distances and reconstruction of phylogenetic trees from microsatellite DNA.Genetics, 144, 189-399.
Tozaki, T, N. Takezaki, T. Hasegawa, N. Ishida, M. Kurosawa, M. Tomita, N. Saitou and H. Mukoyama, 2003. Microsatellite variation in Japanese and Asian horses and their phylogenetic relationship using a European horse outgroup. J. of Heredity 94, 374-380.
Van Haeringen, H., A.T. Bowling, M.L. Scott, J.A. Lenstra. and K.A. Zwaagstra, 1994. A highly polymorphic horse microsatellite locus: VHL20. Anim. Genet. 25, 207.
Vila, C., J.A. Leonard, A. Gotherstrom, S. Marklund, K. Sandberg, K. Linden, R.K. Wayne and H. Ellegren, 2001. Widespread origins of domestic horse lineages. Science. 291, 474-477.
Xu, X. and U. Arnasson, 1994. The complete mitochondrial DNA sequence of the horse, *Equus caballus*: extensive heteroplasmy of the control region. Gene 148, 657-662.

Keyword index

Author index